At Mama's Table

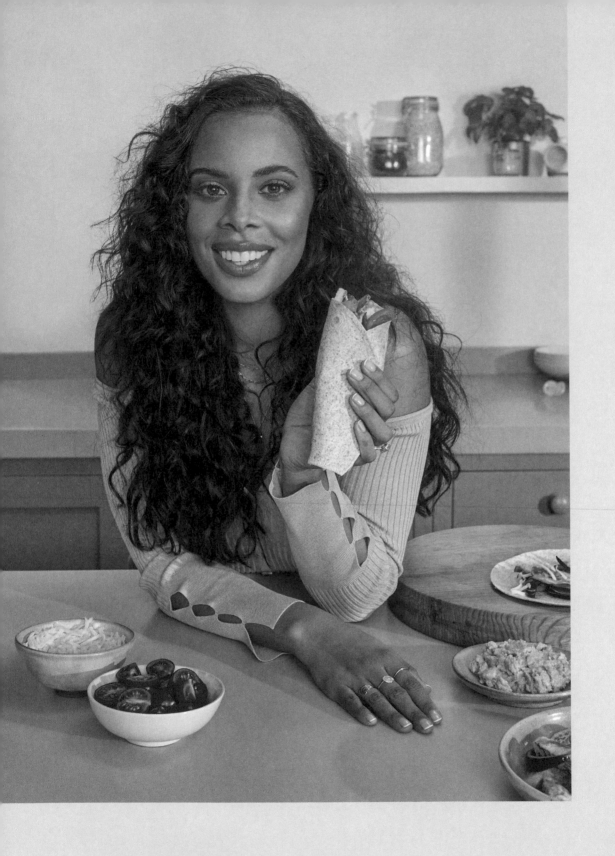

Rochelle Humes

At Mama's Table

Easy & Delicious Meals
From My Family To Yours

Photography by Yuki Sugiura and Karis Kennedy

For my little dream team: Marvin, Alaia, Valle & Blake. My hints clearly weren't enough, so here's a book of all our favourite recipes so that you can cook for me for a change!

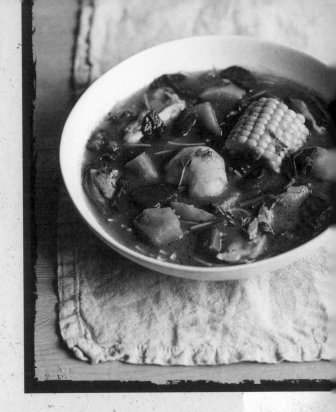

1

Vermilion, an imprint of Ebury Publishing,
20 Vauxhall Bridge Road,
London SW1V 2SA

Vermilion is part of the Penguin Random House group of companies whose addresses can be found at global.penguinrandomhouse.com

 Penguin
Random House
UK

Text copyright © Rochelle Humes
Photography copyright © Yuki Sugiura (food) and Karis Kennedy (portrait)

Commissioning editor: Sam Jackson
Project and copy editor: Dan Hurst
Design and art direction: Nikki Ellis
Nutritional guidance: Julia Wolman
Photography (food): Yuki Sugiura
Photography (portrait): Karis Kennedy
Food styling: Benjamina Ebeuhi
Prop styling: Lucy Attwater

First published by Vermilion in 2021

www.penguin.co.uk

A CIP catalogue record for this book is available from the British Library

ISBN 9781785043758

Printed and bound by Firmengruppe APPL, aprinta druck, Wemding, Germany

The authorised representative in the EEA is Penguin Random House Ireland, Morrison Chambers, 32 Nassau Street, Dublin D02 YH68.

Penguin Random House is committed to a sustainable future for our business, our readers and our planet. This book is made from Forest Stewardship Council® certified paper.

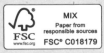

Disclaimer

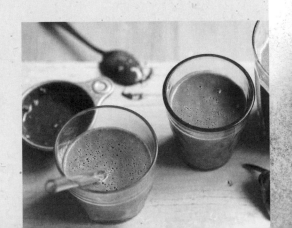

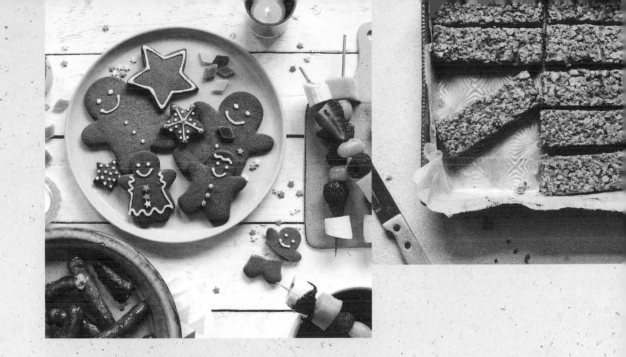

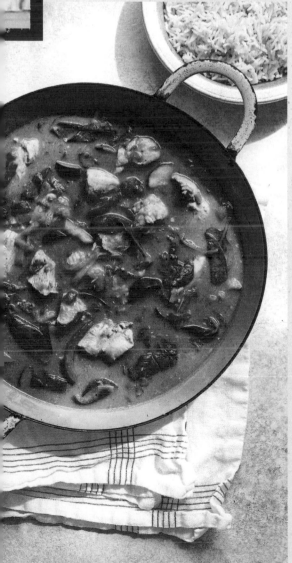

Contents

Introduction

Hi everyone!

Thanks for picking up *At Mama's Table*. The kitchen has always been at the heart of my home. When I was a child and now as a mum, I have always sat down at the end of the day with my family to eat. My husband Marvin and I are big believers in the importance of sitting around the table together and having that quality time as a family. I know too well the busy demands of family life and I always cook one meal for all of us, even if I make a few small changes for the kids. Regardless of how busy we are, Marvin and I will always make it home for dinner, even if it means taking a break from work to come home for a bit or on one of those days when we are playing tag team to look after the kids. Where possible, I try and cook from scratch and I am a huge fan of simple, fresh, and flavoursome meals that everyone can enjoy.

Since I was young, being in the kitchen and cooking a meal for my loved ones has been a kind of therapy for me. I do most of the cooking in our house but that's because I love it and it's how I relax at the end of a long day. Marvin is the drinks guy – that's his strength in the kitchen; making sure everyone has a full glass and the ambiance is good with the right music on! He is also in charge of making brunch at weekends. In our house, we really celebrate food. On special occasions, such Christmas and Easter, our families and friends will come to us and I'll spend a lot of time preparing meals. When we have friends and family over and I cook for them, I am often asked to write my recipes down for them afterwards. I have always said I'll do it, but up until now I have never found the time. Our house is super-busy with Marvin, my two girls Alaia and Valle, and our baby boy Blake, but this year felt like the perfect time to put pen to paper and create a book of recipes that are as suitable for the smallest tummies in the family as they are for the biggest.

I've just been through the weaning journey for the third time and introducing your baby to solid food for the first time can be so exciting. It's natural, especially if you are a first-time mum, to feel nervous when weaning your baby but it is also such an adventure. That feeling that you have cracked it, when your baby has eagerly eaten some broccoli, for example, is the best! I wanted to write this book to show you all how I cook for my family, including the details of how I adapt my recipes for weaning babies. Like many mums, I live a busy lifestyle, so everything – including our family meals – has to slot in with that. I never have time to cook more than once, so I have incorporated guidance in almost all of my recipes so you know how to adapt them to feed weaning babies

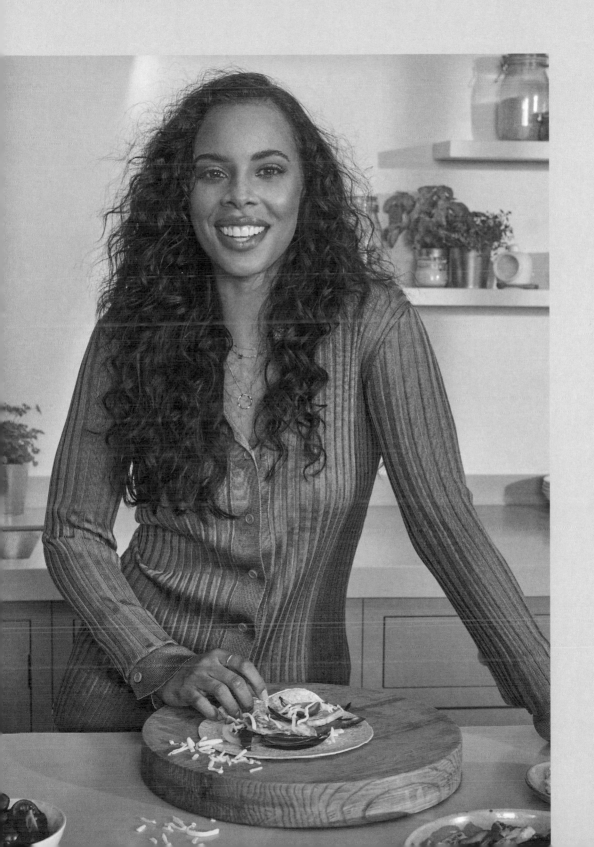

To help you identify the allergens in my recipes I have included symbols on each recipe showing which of the 14 main allergens are included. Use the key below to help identify which allergens are in each recipe:

 Celery

 Crustaceans

 Eggs

 Fish

 Gluten

 Lupin

 Milk

 Molluscs

 Mustard

 Peanuts

 Sesame

 Soya

 Sulphites

 Tree Nuts

and slightly older children, without having to cook for them separately. Cooking in this way means that you'll know that they will be experiencing the full range of flavour, variety, and textures that they need. I've suggested a combination of both purées and baby-led weaning ideas, so you can choose the approach you would like (or do a combination of them, which is what I have always done!). While most of my recipes have this information, there are a small handful that simply aren't suitable for very young children, no matter how much they might enjoy them – sorry kids! This is usually on dessert recipes, where the sugar content is too high for very young tummies, but that just means there's all the more for us parents!

For those who are introducing food to their children for the first time, it is important to make sure your child is ready and to follow NHS guidelines on when to introduce certain foods and potential allergens. When introducing allergens, it is important to do this slowly and one at a time, so you know exactly what food has triggered any reaction that your child may have. To help with this, I have included information on key allergens in all of my recipes (see, left).

All of my recipes are for quick, easy and crowd-pleasing dishes, whether it's food that you can get on the table in next-to-no time and prep-ahead recipes, twists on everyday favourites when you may be stuck in a rut, ideas for food on the move, and occasion dishes that are perfect for dishing up at family celebrations. I have aimed for easy and intuitive recipes, including easy-to-buy supermarket ingredients and no more than ten ingredients in each recipe. I know that busy parents don't have the time to source strange ingredients or follow complicated recipes – if you are anything like me, then you'll like recipes that you can make after a bad night's sleep with your eyes almost shut! There are a couple of slightly more involved and ingredient-heavy recipes, but these are recipes like Pops' Saturday Soup (see page 75), that are so special to us as a family that I simply couldn't write a cookbook without including them.

I believe in a good balance of vegetarian, meat, and fish dishes that are inexpensive, colourful, flavoursome and fun to create. I think sometimes the flavour can be lost when cooking for kids as we try and temper spice or seasoning for younger plates. We are big fans of seasoning in our household and I have introduced my kids to it from early on. Even the simplest of dishes can be elevated with a little careful spicing and my children now love it as much as Marvin and I do. One concession I do make when cooking food for my kids is with salt and pepper, which I try and leave to the end for just the adults at the table rather than seasoning all the way through cooking a meal. Likewise, if a dish calls for stock or salty sauces, such as soy, try and find a low-sodium variety if you are cooking for young children.

My kids are real foodies and I want to encourage them to have a healthy and positive relationship with food. I have always included my girls in cooking and preparing food, whether it is stirring the batter for pancakes, or dipping the homemade chicken or mushroom nuggets into the eggs and breadcrumbs, or baking together. Alaia is the Queen of making dumplings. She is really hands-on and loves to get involved with weighing ingredients and mixing them all together. Valle loves to help, too. I give her a child-safe peeler to help me peel potatoes. I have usually whizzed through a whole bag in the same time she does her one, but she is always very proud of her potato!

Alongside my recipes, I have included feature spreads that give useful tips on how to involve kids and get them excited about food. Whether it is including simple playdate recipes, rainy-day and no-mess baking (where the kitchen doesn't look like a bombsite afterwards), or adding ideas like school pick-up snack heroes, I want to involve the whole family and show everyone how cooking can be fun. Even for the smallest member of the family, exploring food and cooking will build positive associations with food, different textures, and family mealtimes.

I've also included lots of tips and techniques to reduce the legwork for busy parents, including store cupboard essentials, plus ideas about batch cooking and time-saving hacks. The focus of *At Mama's Table* is on simplicity and time, and refreshing culinary imagination, so you can have fun cooking with and for the whole family.

Those who aren't catering for children can enjoy the recipes as they are, without making any changes or subs. When writing this book and when cooking for my family in general it's important to me that this is the food that Marvin and I like to eat, which is one of the reasons I don't make concessions when it comes to flavour. Life's too short to eat bland food!

Enjoy!

Love, Rochelle

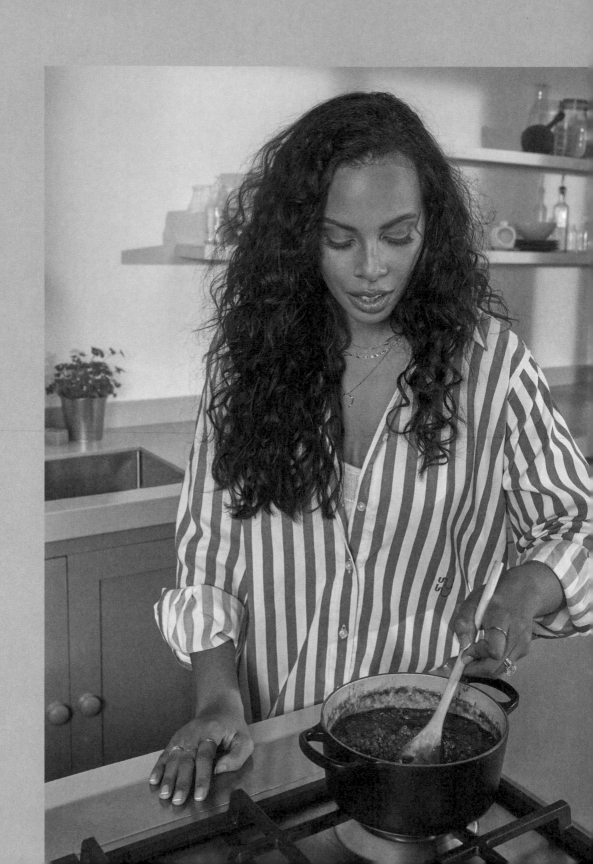

My Top Batch Cooking Tips

Batch cooking is a game-changer because it saves so much time. If it's one of those crazy days where I am handing Marvin the kids to dash to work, or vice versa, there is no better feeling than knowing they are getting a home-cooked meal without one of us having to cook from scratch. If I know I have a busy week ahead and have a relatively chilled weekend, I will think about batch cooking on a Saturday or even first thing on a Monday after I have dropped the kids at school. Here are my top tips.

Make a plan: The most important thing is to plan ahead. Decide what you plan to cook and in what quantity, then buy all the ingredients in one shop. My favourite meals to batch cook are things that are healthy and sustaining, but also popular with the kids. Soups, like my No-Cream, Cream of Tomato Soup (see page 96) and staples like my Veggie (or Beef) Bolognese (see page 126) are always safe bets!

Cook a base sauce: Most dishes start with a base sauce, which can be made ahead and then adapted into different recipes as a way of saving time. For example, a tomato and mince base can be made into Bolognese, chilli, pasta bake, lasagne or cottage pie.

Have the right kit: Do you have loads of containers with no matching lids? We have all wasted hours playing the Tupperware matching game! Decide what containers you will need before you start cooking and set them on the side. I use freezable glass containers, which can be used time and time again.

Always label: When faced with a freezerful of frozen meals, it can be very easy to lose track of what everything is. Pasta sauces, curries, soups, and stews all start to look the same after they are frozen! Label your containers with the contents, date, and anything else that might be useful to know, such as reheating instructions.

Freeze in the right portions: Think about portion sizes when you are packaging things up to freeze. I freeze in slightly smaller portions for Alaia and Valle, then their meals can be defrosted separately on the odd occasion Marvin and I won't be eating with them. If you are weaning, ice-cube trays are perfect for freezing purées or small portions, then you can pop them out and quickly defrost them as you need.

Pack it small: If you are using freezer bags, make sure all the air is squeezed out of the bags, so the meals don't get freezer burn. This also helps save space in your freezer. Also, always make sure all your food is completely cooled before it goes into the freezer.

My Time-Saving Hacks & Tricks

After a busy day at work, everyone wants to spend more time with the family and less time in the kitchen! For many people, cooking can be relaxing and fun, but busy working parents will often be juggling reading, homework, and small children in the afternoons and evenings when everyone is tired. Here are my best hacks:

Plan ahead:
I look at what is in the cupboard and then make a plan for the week based on what I already have to hand. I will then make a list of anything else I need to buy to cook the meals for that week. I also try to fit food around my life, so in the morning after dropping the kids at school, I may decide to do some food prep for dinner> That way I am never left wondering what we are all going to eat five minutes before dinnertime. My kids are starving when they get home from school, so we often eat at around 5pm. Depending on the age of your children and your working hours, it may or may not be possible for you all to sit down together every day, but many of the meals in this book can be made ahead and reheated if mum and dad need to eat their portions later on in the evening.

Prep with food processors:
Good food processors are not cheap but they can make life much easier. Many varieties have blades for chopping and slicing veg, which can take a lot of the hard work out of meal prep and cut down the time considerably.

Arrange your cupboards for convenience:
Always have the tools that you use a lot easily to hand. Items like pans need to be accessible, so I keep mine right under my hob in drawers. I also have everything in my food cupboards stored in separate, clearly labelled glass jars. When I was pregnant with Valle I saw someone had their cupboard organized like this on Instagram and I decided to try it. It is easier to see everything immediately, without having to rummage around.

Use one-pot wonders and slow cookers:
I am such a fan of one-pot cooking (see my One-Pot Veggie, Bean & Quinoa Stew on page 152) . It is just so easy – you can throw everything in and get on with other stuff, whilst stirring occasionally. I also think slow cookers are brilliant and can be used to cook all sorts of dishes.

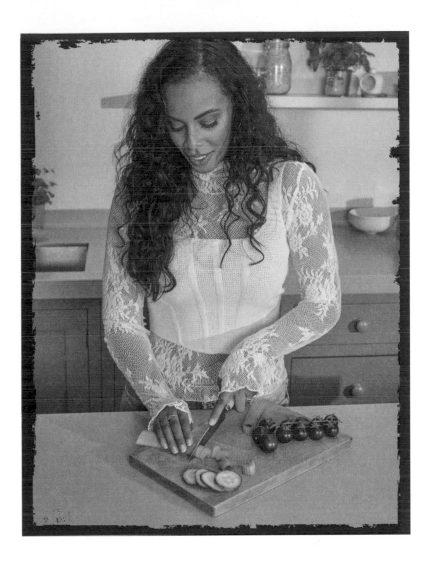

Wash and clear as you go:
There is nothing worse than finishing cooking and being faced with a kitchen looking like a bomb has gone off. I like to cook in stages so that I don't become overwhelmed and always try to clear the sides and wash up or load the dishwasher as I go.

Chop like a pro:
Speed up cooking by cutting veggies with a sharp knife – just make sure you keep them out of the way of any small hands! If your knifes need a sharpen, you can buy knife-sharpening steels relatively cheaply, and a newly sharpened knife is much quicker and safer than trying to chop with a dull, blunt one, which could easily slip and needs an excess of pressure to use. Marvin's dad is a chef and he chops so fast that his hands are a blur!

My Money-Saving Tips

There are loads of smart ways to save money when you cook. One of the main ways is to cook food from scratch. This is just something I try to do every day, though I won't pretend that the odd store-bought chicken nugget doesn't make an appearance on the kids' plates! My other top tips for watching the pennies when you plan your meals for the week are listed below.

Multiple uses: Often one ingredient can cross multiple meals, so, say you're cooking a roast chicken for Sunday lunch and have some leftover, this could make a chicken salad or a soup for lunch the next day (see my Leftover Roast Chicken & Veggie Soup on page 94). Never throw anything away – if you can't use it in the next few days, freeze it instead. Chunky soups and stews can use loads of different veg, so chuck in whatever you have at the back of the fridge.

Buy dry and frozen: Dried beans and lentils are much cheaper than using the canned versions. Also always have some frozen veggies in the freezer. They come pre-chopped, so are easy to use and are actually really healthy – they are picked at their peak and frozen immediately, so are packed with nutrients. When I am batch cooking, I sometimes won't use double the meat or fish to make double the recipe, but will bulk my stews, casseroles, and pasta sauces by increasing the cheaper ingredients instead, such as veggies, lentils and beans.

Go local: Many markets and farm shops sell cheaper fruit and veggies that are locally grown and in season. Even veggies that have been 'marked down' or are wonky can be made into great-tasting soups, casseroles, and pasta sauces. I also go to the local fishmonger and butcher, where the meat and fish are often cheaper and better quality than in the supermarkets. It's also always good to show the small businesses in your local area some love.

Do your food shop online: I do a big cupboard shop online once a week and will buy all my basics like pasta, rice, bread, and milk. I find ordering food online means I stick to the plan I have made for the week. Sometimes, when I am in the supermarket, I can find myself becoming distracted and buy things just because they are on offer or that catch my eye. Never go into the shops on an empty stomach – I always end up loading up my trolley with things that I don't need!

Get organized: I'm obsessed with keeping my storecupboards organized. By keeping glass jars of staples like oats, pasta, and rice, I can easily see what I am running low on, so I can stock up but not order duplicates of things when I don't need them.

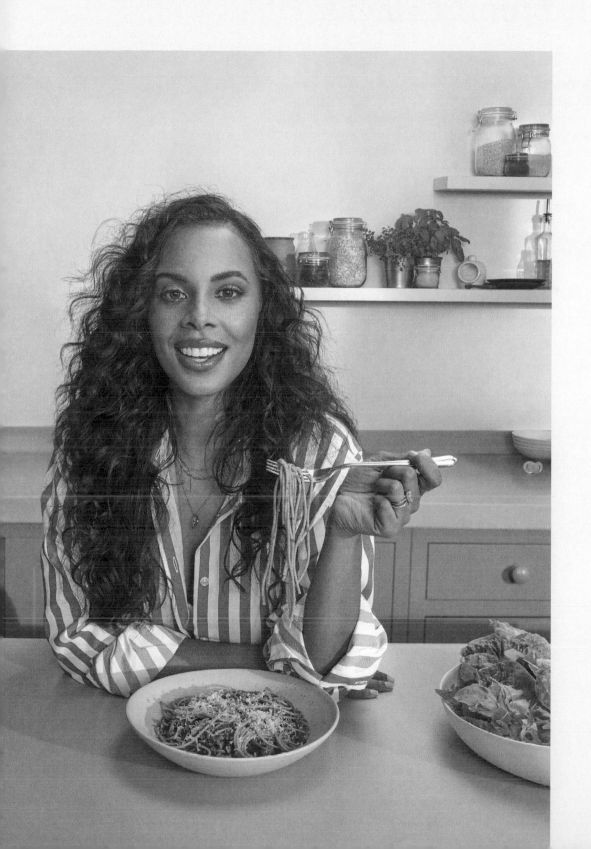

My Freezer Hacks

Freezing food is one of the best ways to make food go further and last much longer, saving time and money. My freezer is packed with easy stuff for the kids and always has a spare loaf of bread for toast. Use the tips below to make sure that you're getting the most out of your freezer, as it really can be your best friend in the kitchen!

Can you freeze it?: There are loads of food items that you can freeze that you may not have thought about. As well as the obvious stuff, we always freeze milk as we seem to go through it so quickly. You can also freeze cooked pasta and rice; it is so easy to cook too much and this means that it won't be wasted.

Jazz it up: I freeze slices of cucumber in blocks and, if you use filtered water, it looks like you have a floating cucumber. The kids love it and I also adore it in a gin and tonic at the end of the day after I've put the kids to bed. Alaia and Valle also like popping frozen blueberries into their drinks to make them more exciting.

Freeze veggies: As well as buying plenty of ready-frozen veg, if you have vegetables in the back of your fridge that you need to use up, they can be part-cooked and then kept in the freezer to save them going off. I blanch or steam them until about half-cooked. This means that when they are defrosted later they will not go soggy.

Fill it up: Did you know your freezer actually runs more efficiently when it is full? I go through my fridge once a month and rotate the contents so the stuff at the front is what needs using up first. This means that nothing gets lost at the back of the freezer and everything is eaten before it goes off. When packing the freezer, I always make sure the most recent batches go to the bottom of the pile, so nothing gets wasted. Make sure everything is labelled. If you want, you could have a list stuck to the door of what is in your freezer that you can add to or cross off as you go.

Get stacking: I love using square and rectangular containers that are great for stacking in the fridge or freezer. If you use freezer bags, ensure there is no air in them and you can lay them flat on top of each other. You can always use your own shelving or storage bins - I always look at Pinterest for ideas.

Basic Equipment

The sky's the limit when it comes to gadgets and equipment, and I must admit, I'm a bit of a kitchen-gadget addict. I find having the right tool for the job makes things so much easier. This list is what I like to have on hand in my kitchen, but is by no means a must-have list for cooking. I put the stuff I use most regularly in the cupboards closest to the hob so I am not endlessly trekking around the kitchen.

Baking:
- Baking dishes
- Cake tins
- Cookie cutters
- Mixing bowls
- Pie dish
- Rolling pin
- Sieve
- Wire rack

Electronics:
- Blender
- Electric Whisk
- Electronic scales
- Food processor
- Juicer
- Slow cooker
- Stand mixer
- Stick blender
- Toastie-maker

Food Preparation and Storage:
- Airtight storage containers
- Can opener
- Good scissors
- Grater
- Knife set
- Measuring jugs
- Mixing bowls
- Non-slip chopping boards
- Oven mitts
- Peeler
- Potato masher (I also have a potato ricer, which is great)
- Salad spinner
- Spatulas
- Whisk
- Wooden spoons

Pans and Oven Dishes:
- Casserole dish
- Colander
- Non-stick frying pan
- Roasting tins
- Set of saucepans
- Sheet pans or baking sheets
- Wok

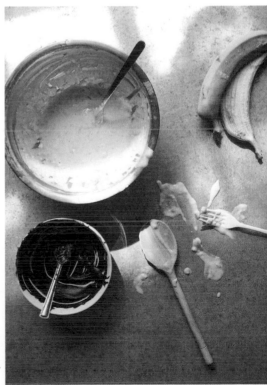

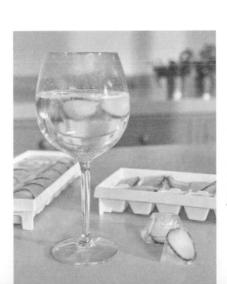

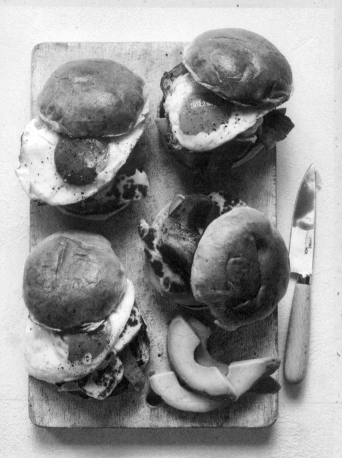

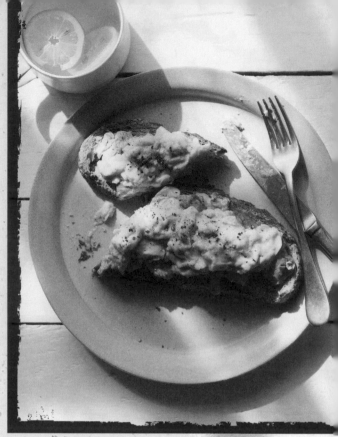

The most important meal of the day!

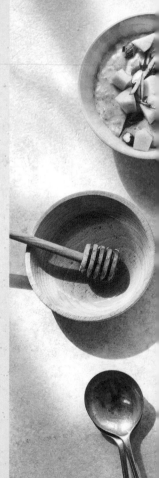

I always like to see the kids go to school set up well for the day. Whether you are looking for something to take some time over on a lazy weekend morning or a filling, grab-and-go option, get your day off to a good start with my breakfast and brunch recipes. Weekdays can be hectic, so some of the recipes, such as my Peanut Butter Overnight Oats (see page 31) or Banana & Berry Layer Pots (see page 41) can be made the night before. We love spending time eating and cooking together at the weekend and Marvin, who hardly ever cooks, will often cook brunch on a Saturday, so my favourite weekend-worthy brunch options are included here, too.

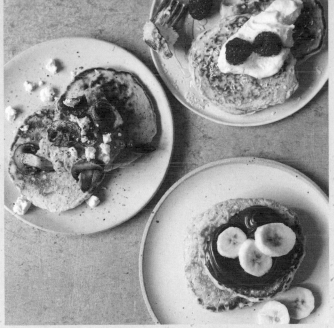

Weekends mean pancakes!

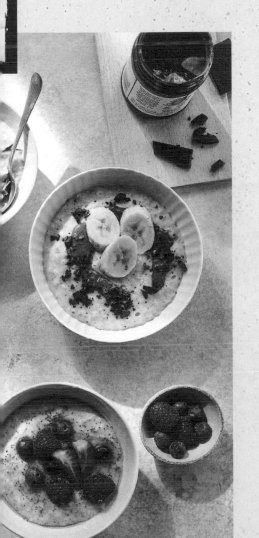

Breakfast & Brunch

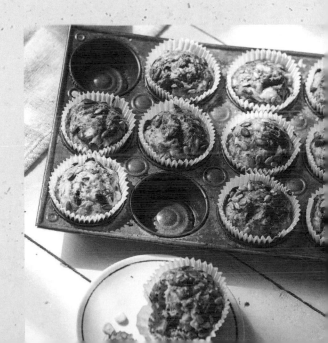

Baked Dippy Eggs

Prep: 5 minutes
Cook: 15 minutes
Serves 4

1 tbsp olive oil
100 g/3½ oz cherry tomatoes, quartered
125 g/4½ oz courgette, grated
50 g/3 oz sliced, honey-roast ham (optional), roughly chopped
100 g/3½ oz frozen spinach
1 x 400 g/14 oz can chopped tomatoes
4 large eggs
40 g/1½ oz feta cheese, crumbled
1 tbsp snipped fresh chives
sea salt and freshly ground black pepper
4 slices wholemeal bread
butter, for spreading
½ avocado, sliced, to serve

For first-stage weaning:
Crack the eggs into the pan with the fried cherry tomatoes and courgettes and cook, stirring until firm and scrambled. Serve the egg-and-veg scramble with soldiers alongside.

For older children:
For older children, simply omit the seasoning before you bake the eggs in the oven.

This rustic recipe is easy to prep, only takes minutes to cook, and the kids always love dipping their soldiers into the egg! I enjoy cooking with eggs because they contain so many key nutrients that the kids need, plus I've sneaked some veggies, including spinach, courgettes, and tomatoes, into this recipe.

Preheat the oven to 200°C/400°F/gas mark 6 and set 4 ramekins on a baking sheet.

Heat the olive oil in a non-stick frying pan over a medium heat, then add the cherry tomatoes, courgette, and ham, if using. Cook, stirring continuously, for 4 minutes until the veg has started to soften. Add the spinach and chopped tomatoes to the pan and stir to combine. Bring the mixture just to the boil, then reduce the heat and leave to simmer for another 5 minutes.

Divide the mixture equally between the ramekins, then crack an egg on top of the tomato mixture in each ramekin, being careful not break the yolks. Top each egg with a quarter of the crumbled feta and a sprinkling of chopped chives. Season the grown-up portions with salt and pepper, then transfer the baking sheet with the ramekins to the oven and leave to cook for 5 minutes until the egg whites are set but the yolks still runny.

While the eggs are in the oven, toast and butter the bread and cut the slices into soldiers. Serve the baked eggs hot with the sliced avocado and buttered soldiers alongside for dipping.

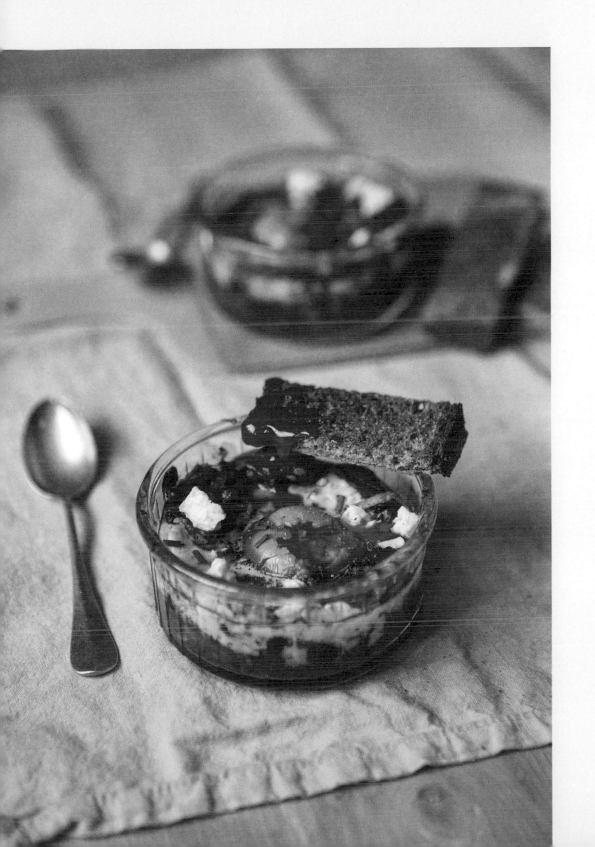

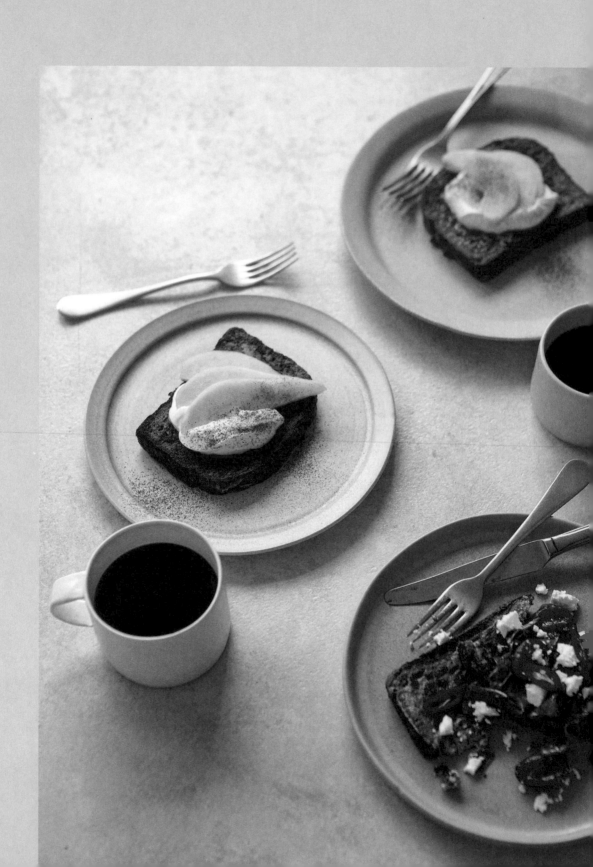

French Toast – Two Ways

French toast is a real favourite in our household as it is so quick and easy to make, yet feels comforting and luxurious. It is also really versatile, so never gets boring. I have suggested two toppings – a sweet one (we love the warmth of the cinnamon in this) and a savoury one, with feta, spinach, and vine tomatoes. I have suggested optional chilli – Marvin and I always add loads to ours!

Prep: 5 minutes
Cook: 8-10 minutes
Serves 4

2 large eggs
50 ml/2 fl oz semi-skimmed milk
4 thick slices wholemeal bread
4 tsp olive oil
4 tsp room temperature unsalted butter

For the cinnamon and pear option:
½ tsp ground cinnamon
2 ripe pears (approx. 300 g/11 oz), peeled
2 tbsp caster sugar, to serve
250 g/9 oz natural yoghurt, to serve

WITH CINNAMON AND PEAR...

Crack the eggs into a wide, shallow bowl, then add the milk and cinnamon and whisk together until well combined. Grate the flesh from 1 of the pears and finely chop or slice the other, discarding the cores from both. Set the chopped or sliced pear aside for later, then add the grated pear to the egg and milk mixture and mix again to combine.

Working with 1 slice of bread at a time, lay the bread flat in the egg mixture and leave to soak for 1-2 minutes, then turn the bread and soak the other side.

While the bread is soaking, place a non-stick frying pan over a medium heat and add 1 teaspoon each of olive oil and butter. Once the pan is hot and the butter has melted, lift the bread, allowing any excess egg mixture to drip back into the bowl, then lay it flat in the pan. Cook for 3-4 minutes until crisp and golden, then flip the bread and cook the other side. Once the bread is cooked, set it aside on a plate while you repeat the process with the remaining slices.

Once all the slices are cooked, divide the French toast between serving plates and serve sprinkled with caster sugar and with a dollop of natural yoghurt and a spoonful of chopped pear on the side.

Continued overleaf...

For the tomato, spinach and feta
  option:
100 g/3½ oz cherry tomatoes
handful of baby spinach
100 g/3 ½ oz feta cheese, to serve
½ red chilli, to serve (optional)

For first-stage weaning:
Cut the French toast into small
batons before serving. If serving
the savoury variation, cut the
tomatoes into quarters and omit
the chilli from the dish.

For older children:
If you are serving the savoury
variation of this dish, cut the
cherry tomatoes into halves or
quarters before serving as they
can present a choking hazard.

WITH TOMATO, SPINACH AND FETA...
Prepare and cook the French toast as described in the
sweet variation on the previous page, omitting the
cinnamon and pear from the egg mixture.

Once all the slices are cooked, return the pan to the
heat and add the cherry tomatoes and spinach and
cook, stirring, for 2–3 minutes until the tomatoes are
just starting to split and the spinach has wilted.

Divide the French toast between serving plates and
spoon over the spinach and tomatoes. Crumble
the feta cheese over the top and spoon over some
chopped red chilli, if using. Serve hot.

Sweet & Savoury Pancakes

We always have pancakes on family birthdays and, if I have any left over, I will either freeze them or put them in the fridge for an after-school snack. Here, I have suggested two sweet and one savoury topping. Our favourite is raspberry and coconut, but I make the banana and chocolate spread option on special days. One quantity of any of the topping recipes makes enough for all of the pancakes, so scale them down if you want to mix and match!

To make the pancakes, add the oats, egg, milk and flour to a large bowl and whisk until well combined. Place a non-stick frying pan over a medium heat and add 1 tablespoon of the coconut oil. Once the oil is hot and melted, swirl it around the pan, then add a ladleful of the pancake batter to the pan to form an 8 cm/3¼ inch pancake. Repeat the process by adding another 2–3 ladlefuls of batter to the pan, ensuring the edges of the pancakes do not touch. Leave to cook for 2 minutes, then carefully flip the pancakes and cook on the other side for 1 minute more until puffed up and lightly golden. Transfer the cooked pancakes to a plate lined with kitchen paper and keep them warm while you repeat the process with the remaining oil and batter.

Once all of the pancakes are made, divide them between serving plates and add the toppings of your choice (see below and overleaf).

FOR THE RASPBERRY AND COCONUT TOPPING:
Spoon the yoghurt over the pancakes, dividing it equally between the serving plates, then dot the raspberries over. Sprinkle with the desiccated coconut and finish each plate with a drizzle of agave syrup, to taste.

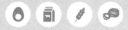

Prep: 5 minutes
Cook: 5–10 minutes (depending on which topping you choose)
Serves: 6–8 pancakes, serving 2–4 people

4 tbsp porridge oats
1 large egg
125 g/4½ oz self-raising flour
125 ml/4½ fl oz semi-skimmed milk
2 tbsp coconut oil

For the raspberry and coconut topping:
125 g/4½ oz fresh raspberries
4 tbsp unsweetened desiccated coconut
agave syrup, for pouring

Continued overleaf...

For the banana and chocolate topping:
4 tbsp chocolate and hazelnut
  spread
2 bananas, peeled and sliced
250 g/9 oz natural yoghurt
handful of toasted, chopped nuts
  (almonds, hazelnuts and pecans
  work well), to garnish

For the mushroom, avocado and feta topping:
1 tbsp olive oil, plus extra for drizzling
handful of chestnut mushrooms,
  sliced
1 garlic clove, finely sliced
1 avocado, peeled and stoned
30 g/1 oz feta cheese
sea salt and freshly ground black
  pepper
chilli sauce, to serve (optional)

For first-stage weaning:
Cut the cooked pancakes into
small batons and serve with
sticks or wedges of fresh fruit
and natural yoghurt, or blend the
fruit into the yoghurt for added
sweetness.

For older children:
Serve the pancakes and toppings
as they as they are, omitting the
nuts if you have any concerns
about allergies.

FOR THE BANANA AND CHOCOLATE TOPPING:
Spoon the chocolate and hazelnut spread over the pancakes,
dividing it equally between the serving plates, then top with
the sliced bananas and a spoonful of natural yoghurt. Scatter
over the toasted nuts, and serve.

FOR THE MUSHROOM, AVOCADO AND FETA TOPPING:
Heat the olive oil in a non-stick frying pan over a medium
heat, then add the sliced mushrooms and garlic, and cook,
stirring occasionally, for 5 minutes.

While the mushrooms are cooking, put the avocado flesh in
a bowl and mash with a fork. Season with salt, pepper and
a drizzle of olive oil, to taste, then spoon over the pancakes.
Spoon the garlicky mushrooms over the avocado and
crumble over the feta cheese. Serve hot, with chilli sauce
alongside for drizzling, if you like.

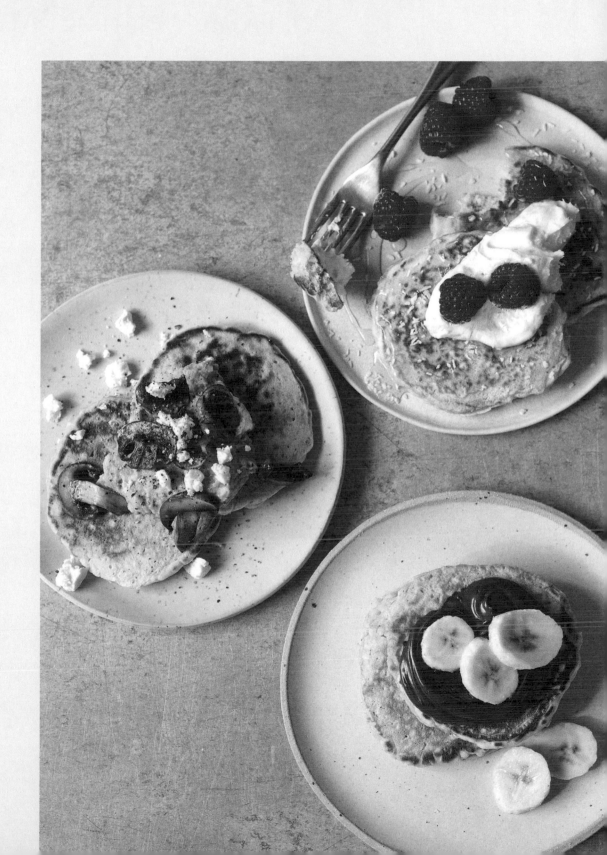

Porridge – Three Ways

Prep: 2 minutes
Cook: 10 minutes
Serves 4

160 g/5¾ oz porridge oats
300 ml/10 fl oz milk
300 ml/10 fl oz water

For the banana, chocolate and peanut butter topping:
2 ripe bananas, peeled and sliced
4 tbsp almond butter
10 g/¼ oz dark chocolate, chopped or grated

For the mixed berry topping:
handful of mixed fresh berries (blueberries, strawberries and raspberries all work well)
poppy seeds, to sprinkle
honey, to drizzle

For the apple, pear and nut topping:
1 apple, peeled and grated
1 pear, peeled and roughly chopped
handful of toasted almonds
pinch of ground cinnamon

For first-stage weaning:
Omit the toppings, but mash sliced bananas or berries into the porridge before serving.

For older children:
Older children can have this with any of the toppings, though always be mindful of allergies and ensure that any fruit is chopped up nice and small to avoid choking hazards.

Porridge is a high-fibre and deliciously warming breakfast choice. We mix up toppings to make it more interesting and here are some of my favourites. The kids love berries, and the mixed-berry version with poppy seeds is one of our go-to toppings, particularly in late summer, when these fruits are in season. The banana, chocolate, and nut butter topping is a special treat for weekends and special days. One quantity of any of the topping recipes makes enough for all four bowls of porridge, so scale them down if you want to mix and match!

Put the oats, milk and water in a medium, non-stick pan and place over a medium heat. Bring the mixture to the boil, then reduce the heat to a gentle simmer and cook, stirring occasionally, for 5–6 minutes until the oats have absorbed the liquid and the porridge is soft and creamy. If the porridge becomes too dry, loosen with a splash more milk. Divide the mixture between serving bowls and add your choice of toppings to each.

FOR THE BANANA, CHOCOLATE AND PEANUT BUTTER TOPPING:
Divide the sliced banana between the 4 bowls of porridge, then drizzle over the almond butter and sprinkle with a little chopped or grated chocolate.

FOR THE MIXED BERRY TOPPING:
Chop any larger berries into halves or quarters, then divide the berries between the bowls of porridge. Sprinkle each bowl with some poppy seeds, then drizzle over a little honey.

FOR THE APPLE, PEAR AND NUT TOPPING:
Divide the grated apple and chopped pears between the bowls of porridge, then scatter over the toasted almonds and finish each bowl with a pinch of ground cinnamon.

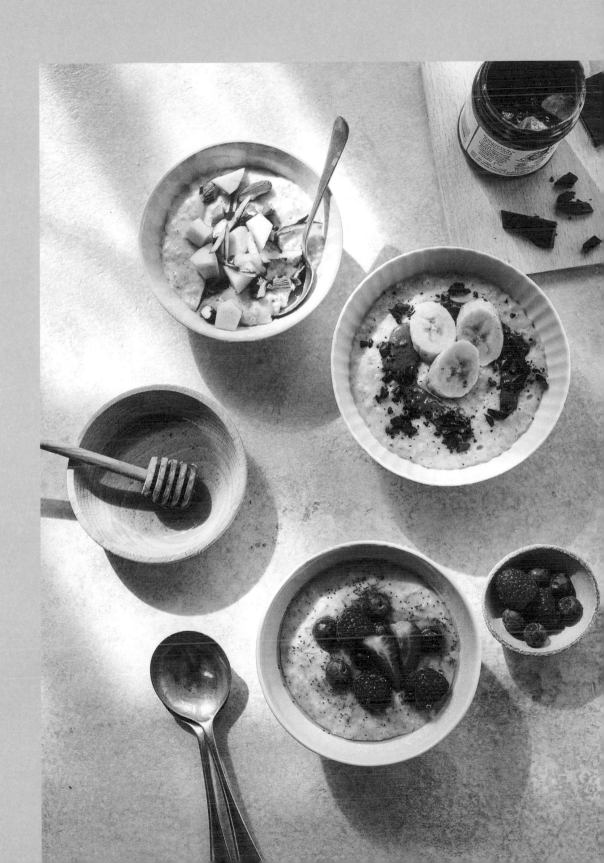

Granola Pots

Prep: 5 minutes
Cook: 25 minutes
Serves 4 (with a little granola
leftover for another day)

200 g/7 oz mixed nuts (almonds,
pecans and hazelnuts work well),
roughly chopped
450 g/1 lb porridge oats
100 g/3½ oz mixed seeds (sesame,
pumpkin and sunflower seeds work
well)
3 tbsp olive oil
125 ml/4 fl oz clear honey or maple
syrup
100 g/3½ oz mixed dried fruit
(raisins, sultanas, dried cherries
and dried cranberries work well)
400 g/14 oz natural yoghurt
150 g/5 oz fresh berries

For first-stage weaning:
You should not introduce honey
into your child's diet until they are
at least 12 months old, and dried
fruits can be hard to chew and
present a choking hazard for very
young children. Blend some fresh
berries with a little yoghurt and
serve it as a purée.

For older children:
Whole nuts are not suitable for
children under five, due to the
risk of choking, so omit them or
substitute for chopped nuts when
feeding preschoolers.

Who doesn't love granola? This homemade version is
great for a speedy breakfast because it is easy to make
ahead and store. These pots are also really nutritious
because they are packed with nuts, seeds and berries,
which are full of healthy fats, protein, fibre, vitamins
and minerals, plus they taste amazing! Kids will love
the fact that they each have a separate pot and, this
way, you can easily store them in the fridge for a
couple of days.

Preheat the oven to 160°C/325°F/gas mark 3 and line a large
baking sheet with greaseproof paper.

Put the chopped nuts, oats and seeds in a large bowl,
then add the oil and honey or maple syrup and stir until
well combined. Tip the mixture onto the prepared baking
sheet and spread out evenly. Transfer to the oven and bake
for 15 minutes, then remove from the oven, give the mixture a
stir to ensure that everything is cooking evenly and return to
the oven for another 10–15 minutes until fragrant and golden
brown. Set aside to cool.

Once the granola has cooled, pour it into a large jar or bowl,
add the mixed dried fruit and stir to combine. Measure out
75 g/3 oz of the granola and set the remainder aside in an
airtight container to use on another day.

To assemble the granola pots, layer the granola and
natural yoghurt in 4 small glasses and finish with a layer
of fresh berries.

Peanut Butter Overnight Oats

Overnight oats are a fab option to make the night before if you know the morning is going to be a huge rush. They're easy, taste delicious, and are really filling, as well as being a great source of fibre and slow-release energy. Marvin is crazy for peanut butter, so this is one of his favourite breakfasts. If you have mixed seeds and nuts in the cupboard, they make an extra-crunchy, nutritious and tasty topping

The evening before you want to serve them, put the oats, 400 ml/14 fl oz of the milk and 1 tablespoon of the peanut butter in a bowl or container with a lid and stir to combine. Cover and leave in the fridge overnight.

The next morning, add the cinnamon and the remaining 100 ml/3½ fl oz of milk to the oat mixture and stir to combine. Spoon the oats into serving bowls and top each with a spoonful of natural yoghurt, fresh berries or grated or chopped fruit of your choice, a drizzle of honey, the remaining peanut butter and a scattering of seeds or chopped nuts, if using.

Prep: 5 minutes
Serves 4

200 g/7 oz rolled oats
500 ml/18 fl oz semi-skimmed milk
  (or dairy-free alternative)
2 heaped tbsp peanut butter
½ tsp ground cinnamon
100 g/3½ oz natural yoghurt
150 g/5 oz fresh berries or grated
  or chopped fruit of your choice
clear honey, to drizzle
2 tbsp mixed seeds or chopped nuts
  (optional)

For first-stage weaning:
Serve the oats simply topped with a little grated apple or mashed banana. Honey is not suitable for children under 12 months.

For older children:
Serve the oats as they are, omitting the peanut butter and nuts if you are concerned about allergies. Ensure that any fruit or berries are chopped small enough not to pose any choking hazard.

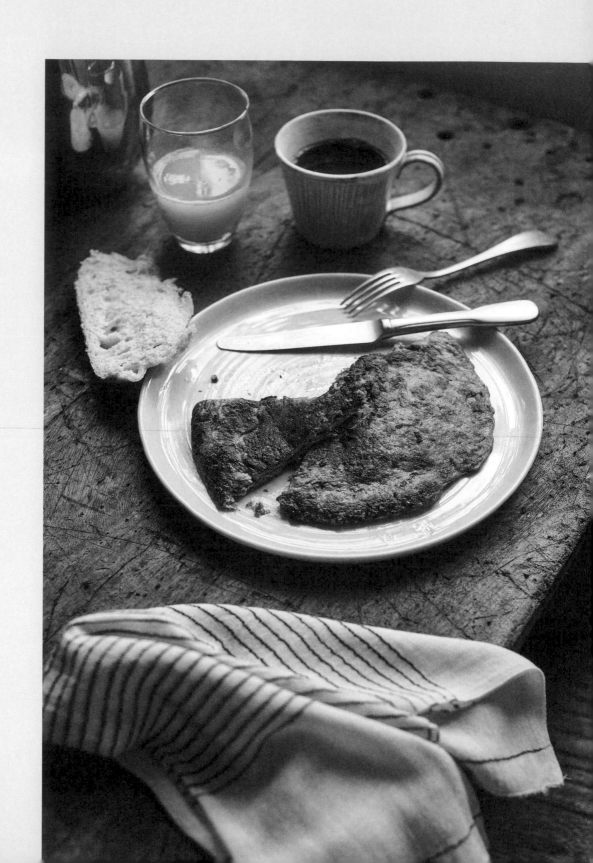

Sweet Potato, Kale & Cheddar Omelette

This is my twist on a classic omelette. For this, you will either need a cooked sweet potato or, to save time, you could peel and grate a raw sweet potato into the bowl when you combine the ingredients. This is also a great way to eat kale, which can sometimes be bitter but is loaded with goodness, and when combined with the sweet potato and cheese, is delicious.

If you do not have any pre-cooked sweet potato, preheat the oven to 200°C/400°F/gas mark 6, place the raw sweet potato on a foil-lined baking sheet and transfer to the oven for 1 hour until soft. Once cool enough to handle, remove the flesh from the skin and weigh out 150 g/5 oz, reserving the remainder to use another time.

Put the cooked sweet potato in a large mixing bowl and mash with a fork until smooth. Pour the beaten eggs into the bowl, add the kale and grated cheese and season with salt and pepper, then mix well to combine.

Heat ½ tablespoon of the olive oil in a 26 cm/10½ inch, non-stick frying pan over a medium heat. Pour in half of the egg mixture, swirling it around the pan so the base is covered in an even layer. For the first 20 seconds or so, as the eggs start to set, use a fork to pull the set edges of the omelette into the centre, swirling the pan to fill the gaps with more of the raw egg mixture – this will ensure that your omelette cooks more evenly. Leave to cook for a further minute or so until the egg has just set, then work around the edges of the pan with a spatula to loosen the omelette. Once loosened, slide the spatula under one side of the omelette and carefully fold it in half. Slide the omelette onto a plate and keep it warm while you repeat the process with the remaining egg mixture.

Prep: 5 minutes
Cook: 10 minutes, plus baking
  the sweet potato
Serves 4

150 g/5 oz pre-cooked sweet potato,
  peeled or 1 raw sweet potato
8 large eggs, beaten
50 g/2 oz kale
60 g/2¼ oz Cheddar cheese, grated
1 tbsp olive oil
sea salt and freshly ground black
  pepper

For first-stage weaning:
Omit the seasoning and slice the omelette into small wedges before serving.

For older children:
Just omit the seasoning when preparing.

Learning
Through Cookery

Like many of us, the lockdowns of 2020 and 2021 taught me that I'm no natural teacher, but I did discover some fun methods to incorporate learning into cooking and baking. Cooking with my kids is a great way to spend quality time, especially on rainy days, and I've found it great for their creativity and imagination. As well as reading and weighing ingredients and writing lists, there are loads of things you can teach your kids through cooking. Here are just some of the ideas that I have used or plan to use with Alaia and Valle.

Maths Biscuits

How can you make maths fun at home? Add some biscuits and it can become a little more interesting. Younger children may enjoy learning about shapes by using biscuit cutters to cut their dough into 2D shapes like circles and triangles. If you make a batch of around 24 biscuits, there are many things you can do to get the kids to boost their confidence with numbers. Add them and take them away to practise addition and subtraction. Share them out to learn more about division.

Older kids can also learn about fractions, from quarters, thirds, and halves of each biscuit, using icing. Or use the whole batch to describe a third (8/24 biscuits) and then practise adding fractions together. Best of all – everyone gets to eat the biscuits once the activity has been completed!

Alphabet Salad

Younger kids will love trying to make a fruit salad with fruits and vegetables starting with different letters. Start with A and, if your child can name a fruit starting with that letter, such as apple, add that fruit to the bowl. Kids can also practise writing a list as they go if they would like to. See how many different types of fruits they can name. I always add pomegranates, orange and carrots to my salads for the kids, if you are stuck on those letters.

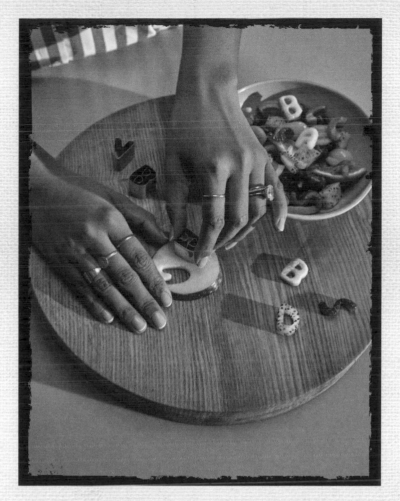

♡ Using alphabet cutters to stamp out letters from the fruit makes this even more impactful.

Mini Science Lab

Cooking involves lots of science ideas – not all science involves fancy labs and lots of different strange materials. As well as seeing what happens when ingredients are mixed together in different quantities, kids can learn about different forms such as solid, liquid, and gases. Explain that when ingredients are put together, they make a mixture. The cake batter starts as a liquid but turns solid after it is heated in the oven. Or chocolate will melt when it is heated. Show them how water can freeze solid or evaporate when heated.

Cheesy Scrambled Eggs with Avocado

Prep: 2 minutes
Cook: 5 minutes
Serves 4

6 large eggs
50 g/2 oz Cheddar cheese, grated
1 tsp olive oil
butter, for frying and spreading
4 slices wholemeal bread
2 ripe avocados, peeled and stoned
sea salt and freshly ground black
    pepper
sauces of your choice, to serve

For first-stage weaning:
Serve the cheesy scrambled eggs unseasoned. Mash the avocado into the toast, slice into soldiers and serve on the side.

For older children:
Older children will enjoy this as it is (though they may like their toast served as soldiers). Omit the seasoning when making the scrambled eggs and pass it to adults separately when serving the meal.

Master the perfect eggs and avo with this recipe. These are two of my favourite foods and this is a great choice for even the fussiest eaters. My kids love avocado, which are full or nutrients and healthy fats, so this recipe always gets their day off to a great start. I try to use wholemeal or seeded bread for extra fibre, but sometimes we will also enjoy this on toasted sourdough.

Crack the eggs into a large bowl, season with salt and pepper, and beat with a whisk or fork until well combined. Add the cheese to the bowl and stir to combine.

Heat the oil and a knob of butter in a non-stick frying pan over a medium heat, then pour in the egg and cheese mixture and cook, breaking the eggs up with a spatula or wooden spoon, for 3–4 minutes until the eggs are scrambled and cooked through, but still silky. Remove from the heat.

While the eggs are cooking, toast and butter the bread and divide the pieces between 4 serving plates. Put the avocado flesh in a bowl and gently mash with a fork, then spoon the avocado over the slices of toast, spreading it out in an even layer.

Spoon the scrambled eggs over the avocado-topped toast and add any seasonings or sauces that you like. Serve hot.

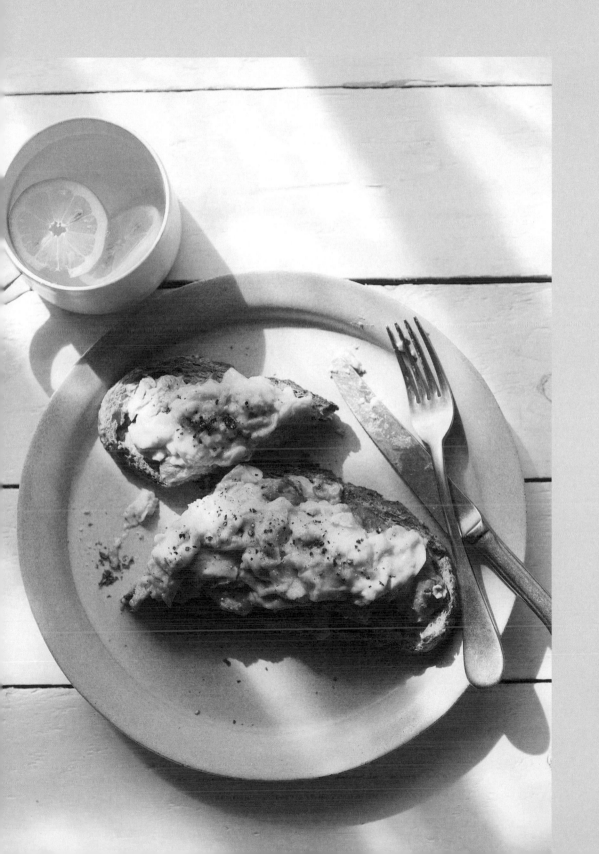

Courgette & Potato Rösti

Prep: 10 minutes
Cook: 20 minutes
Serves 4

1 medium courgette (approx.
 150 g/5 oz), grated
600 g/1 lb 5 oz white potatoes,
 grated
2 tbsp butter
3 tbsp sunflower oil
sea salt and freshly ground
 black pepper
4 large eggs

For first-stage weaning:

Omit the seasoning from the
rösti and cut it into small wedges
for easy holding. Scramble,
rather than fry the egg to serve
alongside.

For older children:

Older children can enjoy this as
it is. You may want to omit the
seasoning and pass it around
separately to the adults when
serving.

This is a bit like hash browns, but this rösti recipe is
much healthier. If you like your rösti extra crispy, make
sure you squeeze the moisture out of the mix as much
as possible, or else it may end up a bit soggy. The kids
will eat these served on their own, but for an extra treat
I have suggested pairing them with fried eggs. Enjoy!

Pile the grated courgette and potatoes onto the centre
of clean tea towel, then bring up the sides to enclose the
vegetables. Working over a sink or large bowl, twist the base
of the tea towel as tightly as you can to remove any excess
water from the courgette and potatoes. Tip the courgette and
potato into a large bowl and season with salt and pepper.

Heat 1 tablespoon each of the oil and butter in a 26 cm/
10½ inch, non-stick frying pan over a medium-low heat.
Tip the courgette and potato mixture into the pan and use a
spatula or wooden spoon to spread it out to the edges in an
even layer. Cook for 2–3 minutes, without touching the pan
to allow the rösti to bond, then give the pan a gentle shake to
ensure the mixture isn't sticking. Continue to cook for another
10 minutes, shaking the pan occasionally until the underside
is crisp and golden.

Using a plate and being careful of the hot pan, carefully
flip the rösti out of the pan so that the uncooked side is
now on the base. Return the pan to the heat and warm the
remaining butter, and another tablespoon of oil, then slide
the rösti back into the pan and cook in the same way for
another 10 minutes until the base is crisp and golden and
the vegetables are tender.

If you have another frying pan, heat the remaining oil over
a medium heat while the rösti is cooking, crack the eggs into
the pan one at a time and fry for 3–4 minutes until the white
is set and the yolk is done to your liking. If you don't have
another pan, slide the cooked rösti onto a plate and keep
it warm while you return the pan to the heat and cook the
eggs. Cut the rösti into quarters and divide between 4 serving
plates, topping each piece of rösti with a fried egg. Serve hot.

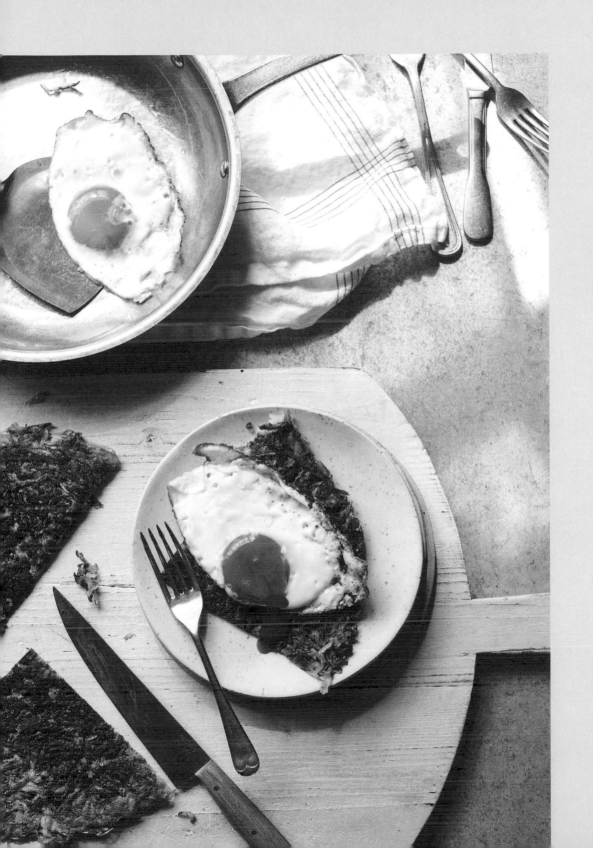

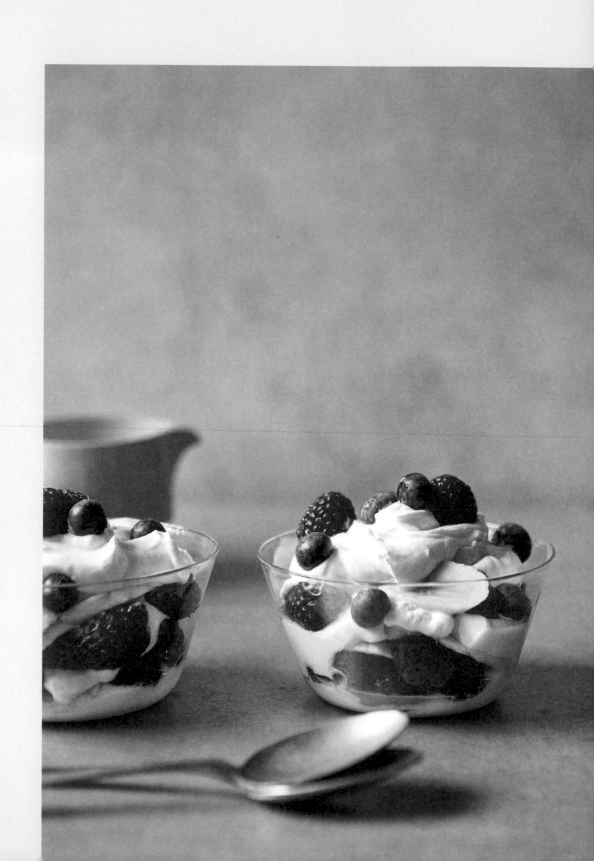

Banana & Berry Layer Pots

This is such a simple recipe but the kids love it. The pots are so fresh and perfect for the summer. Not only do they taste yummy, but they look really pretty! They are ideal for a make-ahead breakfast, so if you are having a busy day, you can grab and go. They are also a fab snack option. I've suggested using natural or Greek yoghurt, though dairy-free or coconut yoghurt would work just as well.

If using strawberries, hull and chop them into bite-sized pieces. Cut any other larger pieces of fruit into bite-sized pieces (smaller raspberries and blueberries can be left whole).

Set 4 small serving bowls or glasses on the counter and put a tablespoon of yoghurt into the base of each. Add a layer of banana slices to each bowl, followed by another layer of yoghurt, then a layer of berries. Continue to layer up the bowls in this way until all of the yoghurt and fruit has been used up. Drizzle a little agave syrup over each bowl and serve.

Prep: 5 minutes
Serves 4

250 g/9 oz strawberries, raspberries
  or blueberries (or a mix of all 3)
1 ripe banana, peeled and sliced
350 g/12 oz Greek or natural yoghurt
2 tbsp agave syrup

For first-stage weaning:
Mash the banana or berries into the yoghurt, then feed to your child or allow them to feed themselves.

For older children:
Chop the fruit into smaller pieces to avoid any potential choking hazards, then stir through the yoghurt.

My Top Weaning Tips

As milestones go, weaning your baby can feel like a big one. It is also exciting – you get to introduce your baby to one of life's greatest pleasures – food! The signs that your baby is ready include when they can stay in a sitting position and hold their head steady, when they start to show more interest in what you are eating, and will happily swallow food that is offered rather than spitting it out. Always talk to your health visitor or check out the guidelines on the NHS website if you are unsure about the right stage to start. There are loads of things that I found made the process easier, here are some of my favourites.

There is no one-size-fits-all:

When I was a first-time mum, I thought there was a 'right' way of doing things, but now I realise we are all just doing our best, and what works for us and our families. When weaning, I like to offer my children homemade purées, just so that I know exactly what they're eating, but I also try and combine it with elements of baby-led weaning. Combining both approaches works for me as it means that my kids are exposed to a range of textures and flavours from a young age, but do whatever works for you.

Don't panic:

Like many mums, I really worried that if my baby had solid food they might choke. It's important to know that gagging is really common when babies start solids and is a natural reflex. It can happen quite often, so it is a good idea to read up on the risks and how to manage it if it does occur, and try not to panic. If you are fearful about choking, one thing I found useful was going on a baby first-aid course, where I learned what to do if my baby got something stuck in its throat, which made me feel much more confident.

Resist cleaning up:

Weaning babies is a messy job and it can be tempting to
hover over your child while they are eating, cloth in hand,
but it's really important for babies to explore, handle and taste
lots of different types of foods, even if a lot of it goes on the floor!
My tip is this: do not clean up until the end of the meal when your
baby has finished eating. Otherwise you will spend the entire time
wiping your child, their chair, and the kitchen floor. If you have
long hair, tie it up and definitely don't wear white! Whenever I
wore light clothes my kids were guaranteed to sneeze their
brightly coloured purées all over me!

Be patient:

When I weaned Alaia, she was a dream and ate everything
that I gave her. Valle, on the other hand, was a whole other story.
I expected her to be the same as Alaia, but, of course, she wasn't,
because each child is unique. Lots of babies take time to get used
to the idea of food, so just go at the pace of your baby and try
not to compare them to others (including your own!).

New tastes one at a time:

It can be easy to get over-excited and want to offer lots of foods
at once, but try to offer your baby only one or two new tastes
every day when you start weaning. Once they are happy with
those, you can move on. This is especially true when introducing
potential allergens (see the list page 8), which need to be introduced
slowly and one at a time so that you can monitor your child for any
allergic reactions.

Halloumi, Bacon, Avo & Egg Breakfast Baps

Prep: 5 minutes
Cook: 10 minutes
Serves 4

1 tbsp olive oil
1 x 225 g/8 oz block halloumi cheese,
    cut into 8 slices
4 rashers smoked streaky bacon
    (optional)
4 large eggs
4 brioche buns or wholemeal wraps
tomato ketchup or brown sauce
    (optional)
1 ripe avocado, peeled, stoned and
    sliced
50 g/2 oz spinach leaves

For first-stage weaning:

Mash some of the avocado with
a little yoghurt or blend with
some spinach leaves to create
a super green purée.

For older children:

For toddlers and pre-schoolers,
cut up pieces of the cooked
egg, halloumi, bacon and
avocado and serve with some
toasted bun for chewing on.
School-age children will enjoy
these as they are.

This recipe is the perfect cure for a bad night's sleep, or
for those mornings when you have had a few too many
drinks the night before! They are delicious served in
fluffy brioche buns, but you could also just throw it all
together in a wrap if you prefer. If you are vegetarian,
just leave out the bacon or use veggie 'bacon' instead.
I've suggested adding ketchup or brown sauce, but you
can add whatever sauce you like.

Place 1 large or 2 smaller frying pans over a medium heat and
add the oil. Once hot, add the sliced halloumi to the pan along
with the bacon rashers, if using. Cook the halloumi and bacon
for 2–3 minutes until nicely golden on the underside, then flip
to cook the other sides. At this point, crack the eggs into the
pan or pans and cook for 2–3 minutes until the whites are set
and the yolks are cooked to your liking. Cooking everything in
this way should ensure all the elements are cooked and ready
at the same time, but if you don't have a pan large enough
or multiple pans, then cook the halloumi and bacon first and
keep them warm while you cook the eggs.

If using brioche buns, slice your buns and spread the bases
with your choice of sauce, then top each with some sliced
avocado and a handful of spinach leaves. Divide the bacon,
eggs and halloumi between the buns and finish with a few
more spinach leaves and an extra squirt of sauce before
adding the bun tops. If using wraps, toast them quickly in the
pan, divide the fillings between the wraps, add a squeeze of
sauce and wrap them up before digging in. Either way, be
prepared to get messy!

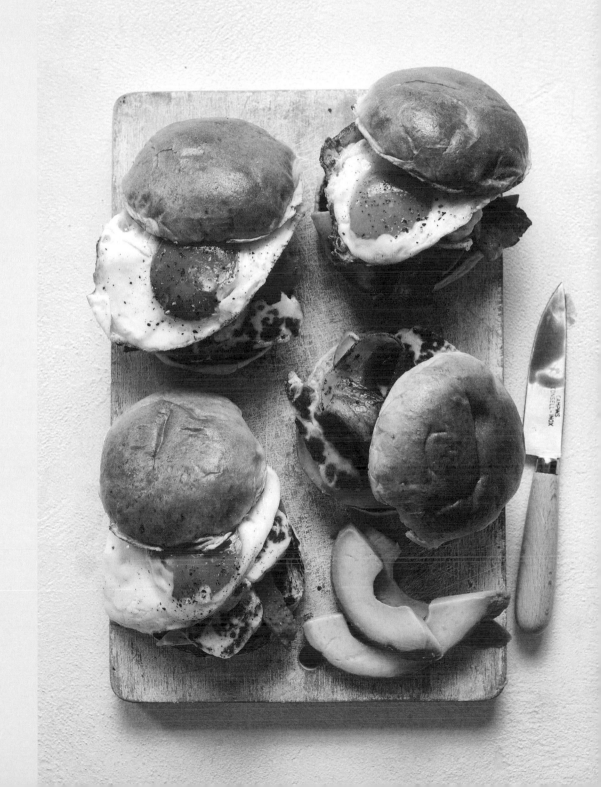

Sweetcorn, Mushroom & Parmesan Muffins

These savoury muffins are packed full of flavour and everyone in the house will love them. It may seem like an odd combination at first glance, but they taste amazing and are packed full of nutrients. They're a great way to get more veggies into the kids from the start of the day, and if they are fussy about cheese with a stronger flavour than Cheddar, this is a fab way to introduce Parmesan. This recipe is a winner!

Preheat the oven to 180°C/350°F/gas mark 4 and line a 12-hole muffin tin with muffin cases.

Put the garlic, mushrooms, sweetcorn, flaxseeds, 30 g/ 1 oz of the Parmesan and 3 tablespoons of the pumpkin seeds in a large bowl, then sift over the flour. Crack the eggs into a separate bowl and beat together with the yoghurt and lemon zest until well combined. Pour the egg and yoghurt mixture into the bowl with the dry ingredients, season with salt and pepper, then stir until everything is just combined.

Spoon the mixture into the prepared muffin cases, splitting it evenly between each case, then sprinkle over the remaining pumpkin seeds and Parmesan. Transfer to the oven to bake for 20–25 minutes until golden, well risen and an inserted skewer comes out clean. Cool for 5 minutes in the tin, then transfer the muffins to a cooling rack and leave to cool completely before serving.

Prep: 5 minutes
Cook: 25 minutes
Makes 12

1 garlic clove, finely grated
150 g/5 oz white mushrooms, roughly chopped
1 x 198 g/7 oz can sweetcorn, drained (165 g/5¾ oz drained weight)
3 tbsp ground flaxseeds
40 g/1½ oz Parmesan, finely grated
4 tbsp pumpkin seeds
150 g/5 oz self-raising flour
3 large eggs
225 g/8 oz natural yoghurt
zest of 1 lemon
sea salt and freshly ground black pepper

For first-stage weaning:
Omit the seasoning from the muffin mixture and leave off the pumpkin seeds when topping the muffins, as they can present a choking hazard. Serve the muffins cut into quarters for easy holding.

For older children:
These can be enjoyed as they are by older children.

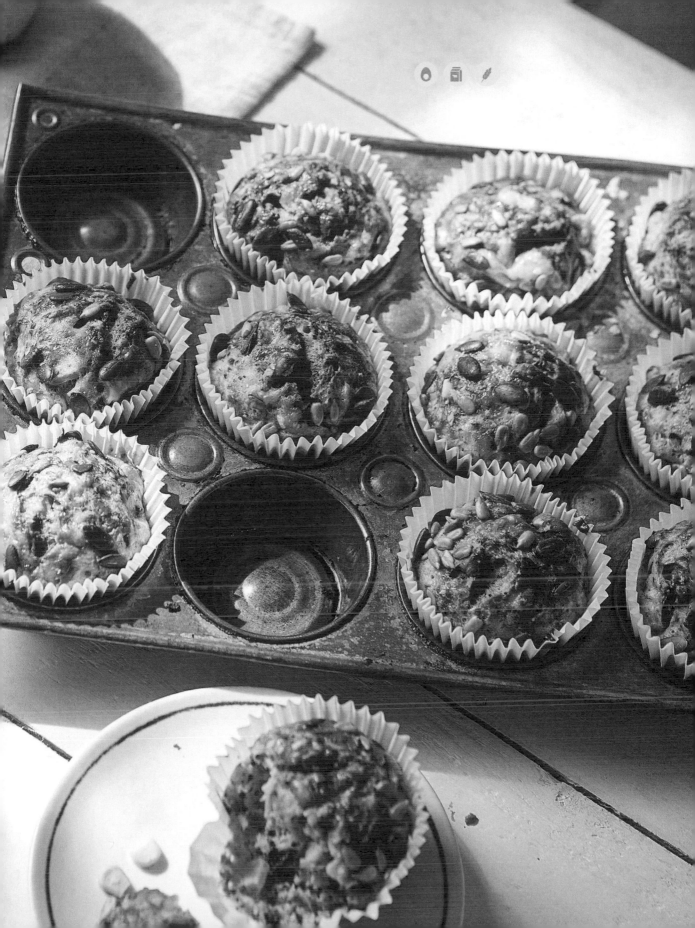

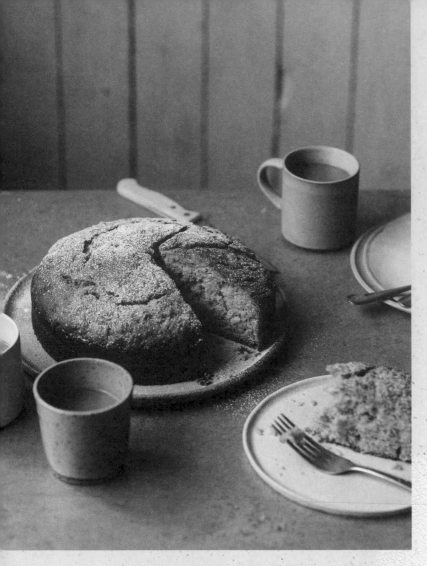

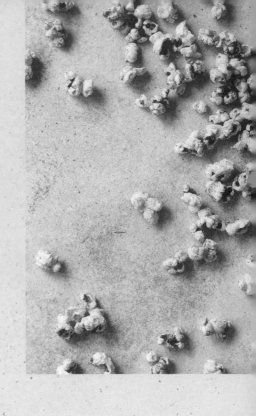

These oaty bars are packed full of energy!

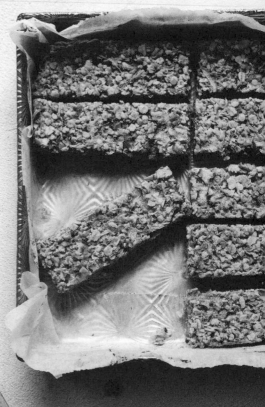

There is nothing more satisfying than the perfect snack. My kids are often in the cupboard at 10am, asking if they can have some sweets and the answer is always no! It's like they are walking around with two stomachs – one for meals and one for snacks. My morning snacks have a healthy spin and are packed full of whole foods and goodness, to give everyone enough energy for the rest of the day. Kids will love ideas like Homemade Trail Mix (see page 61) and Oaty Apple & Pear Bars (see page 66).

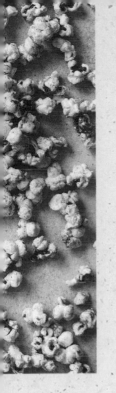

Mid-Morning Snacks

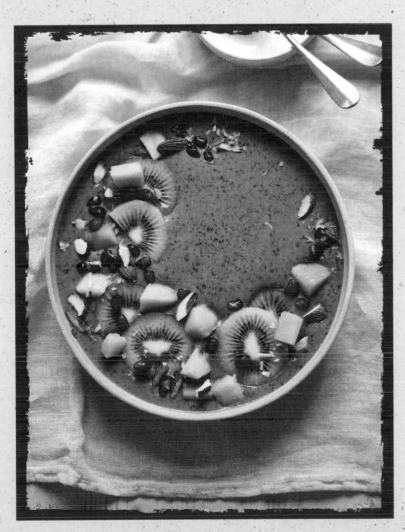

Too pretty to eat! ♡

Blueberry Smoothie Bowl

Prep: 10 minutes
Serves 4

100 g/3½ oz frozen blueberries
2 frozen bananas, peeled and sliced
250 g/9 oz natural yoghurt
1 tbsp ground flaxseed
splash of milk or plant-based milk
  of your choice

For the topping:
4 tbsp natural or dairy-free yoghurt
1 mango, peeled, stoned and cut
  into bite-sized pieces
1 kiwi fruit, peeled and cut into
  bite-sized pieces
60 g/2¼ oz pomegranate seeds
125 g/4½ oz granola or mixed
  nuts, toasted and chopped
agave syrup, for drizzling

For first-stage weaning:
Serve the smoothie bowl without
any of the toppings.

For older children:
For under fives, omit any whole
nuts and the pomegranate seeds,
as these can present a choking
hazard. Otherwise, this can be
enjoyed as it is, just be mindful of
an allergies and ensure that fruit
is chopped up small enough not
to pose a choking hazard.

It might sound strange to serve a smoothie in a bowl,
but this recipe looks beautiful and tastes so fresh and
vibrant. It's thicker than the average smoothie but still
really light and refreshing. You can use any type of milk
that you like to loosen it – Alaia and I love this with oat
milk, but Valle has hers with dairy.

Put the frozen blueberries and bananas in a blender and
blend until smooth, then add the yoghurt and flaxseeds and
blend again until smooth and creamy. If the mixture doesn't
come together, add a splash of dairy or plant-based milk to
help loosen it, then blend again.

Divide the mixture between 4 serving bowls and top each with
a dollop of natural yoghurt, some chopped mango and kiwi,
a sprinkling of pomegranate seeds, a spoonful of granola or
toasted nuts and a drizzle of agave syrup.

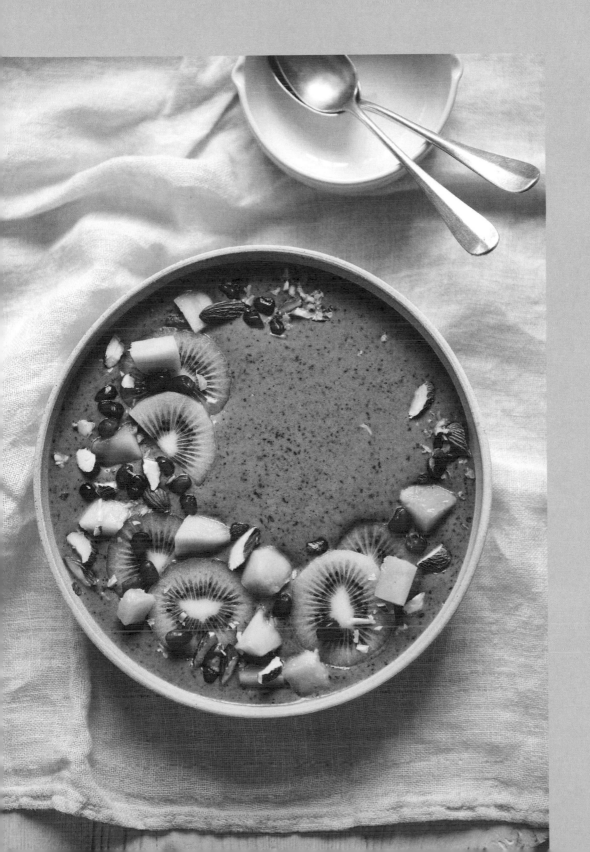

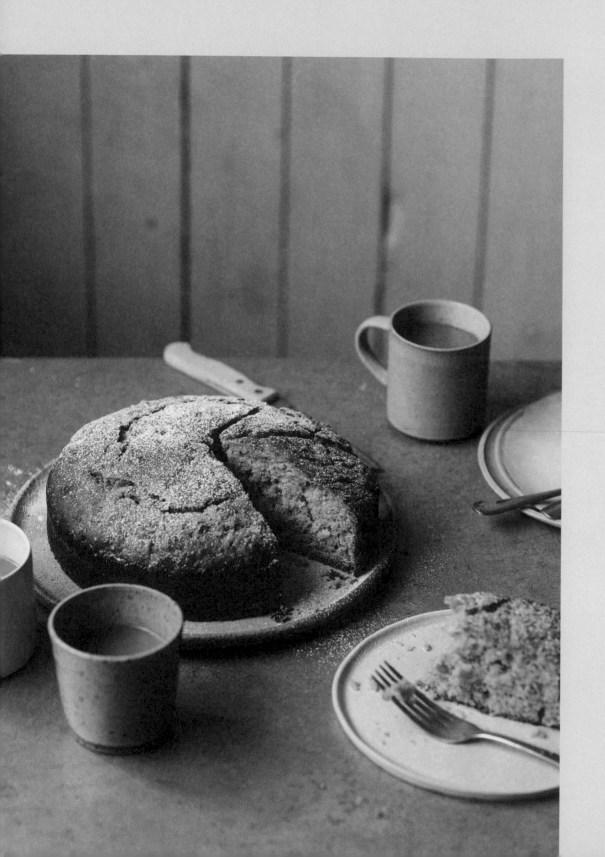

Apple Cake

This cake always gets the thumbs-up from my family. I'll often make this on a Saturday morning and leave it out on the side for everyone to help themselves. It has a really warming and buttery taste, even though it has no actual butter in it. This makes the perfect accompaniment to a morning cup of tea or coffee.

Preheat the oven to 180°C/350°F/gas mark 4 and grease a 20-cm/8-inch cake tin with butter and line the base with greaseproof paper.

Sift the flour, baking powder and cinnamon into a large bowl, then add the grated apples and set aside. Crack the eggs into another bowl and beat together with the sunflower oil, golden caster sugar and vanilla paste until well combined.

Pour the egg mixture into the bowl with the flour and apples and mix with a spatula or wooden spoon until well combined. Pour the mixture into the prepared cake tin and level out the top, then transfer to the oven to bake for 30 minutes until golden, well-risen and an inserted skewer comes out clean.

Leave to cool in the tin for 10 minutes, then turn the cake out onto a wire rack and leave to cool completely. Slice the cake and enjoy with a cup of tea. This will keep well in an airtight tin for a couple of days.

Prep: 15 minutes
Cook: 30 minutes
Serves 12

300 g/10½ oz plain flour
1 tbsp baking powder
pinch of ground cinnamon
2 large apples (approx. 400 g/14 oz), peeled and grated
3 large eggs
160 ml/5½ fl oz sunflower oil
150 g/5 oz golden caster sugar
1 tsp vanilla paste

For first-stage weaning:
Because of the sugar, this is best avoided by children who are under 12 months.

For older children:
Older children can enjoy the cake as it is.

How to Push the Veggies

How do you get kids to eat more veggies? Alaia has always eaten loads of veg, but Valle has been a bit trickier. Thankfully, over time she has improved, but I still sometimes have to disguise vegetables in sauce and use other tricks, including telling her that I always used to eat them as a child. Children (and some adults!) have a preference for sweeter tastes, so getting them to eat more bitter veggies, such as broccoli, can feel like an upward struggle at times. My nieces and nephews often arrive at our house saying they won't eat dinner and then leave having tried something new!

Pair with familiar foods:

What's great about veggies is that there are so many of different varieties and they can be incorporated into your child's favourite meals really easily. Treat foods, such as pizzas, can easily be topped with healthy veg, and I always add loads of peppers and courgettes to tomato sauces and into soups, which you can easily disguise by blending.

Choose a new veggie:

If I have the girls with me and we pop to the shops, I will often suggest that they choose a vegetable or fruit that they don't know and we take it home and do something with it. The more unusual and colourful the fruit or veg the better!

Add some flavour:

Seasoning is a wonderful way of giving vegetables some zing and keeping them interesting. I sometimes roast veggies with a bit of garlic, butter and olive oil and my kids love eating raw veggies like carrots, peppers and celery with dips – see my recipe for Chickpea, Red Pepper & Roasted Butternut Squash Hummus on page 108.

Pretty them up:

I try to make veggies look as appealing as possible by cutting carrots into ribbons or stamping other veg into interesting shapes, such as stars. Sometimes, if I have time, I will even make faces or animals out of veg. Simply making a happy face out of peas is enough to encourage my kids to eat them.

Dish up veggie fries:

All kids love chips! When I cook potato wedges, I also cook other vegetables to create a multicoloured feast. You can make fries out of almost any types of vegetable – just be sure to cut them into the same size so they cook evenly. I like to use carrots, parsnips and courgettes, which are all are easy to do. Other veggies like kale can easily be cooked to make veggie crisps – see my recipes for Crunchy Chickpeas & Kale Crisps on page 56.

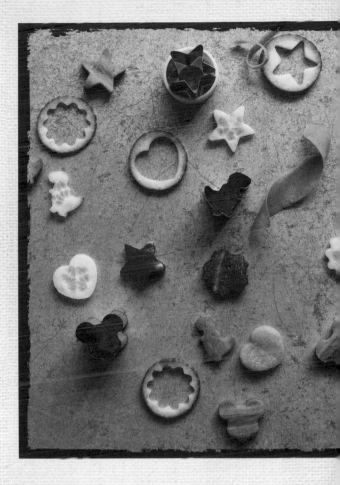

Create veggie people:

Getting your children to play with veg is one of the best ways to get them interested. Creating veggie sculpture people with tomatoes, carrots, cucumbers, broccoli, and cauliflower is really fun. Simply chop up a range of veg and let everyone unleash their creativity using their plate as a canvas. Everyone loves nibbling the arms or head of their new person.

Give them new names:

Your kids might enjoy giving veggies different and fun names, like broccoli 'trees', 'x-ray' carrots, 'surfboard' celery, and cauli 'flowers'. When I serve up broccoli trees, they always seem to go down much better than normal broccoli.

Crunchy Chickpeas & Crispy Kale Crisps

Prep: 5 minutes
Cook: 20–25 minutes
Serves 4

1 x 400 g/9 oz can chickpeas, drained
125 g/½ oz kale, tough stalks removed
1 heaped tsp smoked paprika
2 tbsp mixed seeds (sunflower and sesame seeds work well)
4 tbsp olive oil

For first-stage weaning:
Steam the kale until tender, then blend with some of the chickpeas to make a simple kale hummus.

For older children:
For under fives, omit the chickpeas, as these can present a choking hazard. Older children can enjoy these as they are, though you may want to reduce the amount of paprika to accommodate young taste buds.

This is such an easy and tasty way of getting more veggies into the kids. They taste almost like crisps, but have so many nutritional benefits: chickpeas are a rich source of fibre, vitamins and minerals, whilst kale is loaded with antioxidants. Paprika also gives them a delicious flavour. My kids always devour these, fresh out of the oven.

Preheat the oven to 180°C/350°F/gas mark 4.

Tip the drained chickpeas into a large roasting tin and roll with a sheet of kitchen paper to dry them out. Add the kale to the tray, followed by the paprika and seeds. Drizzle over the olive oil, then use your hands to toss everything together, making sure the kale and chickpeas are nicely coated in the paprika and oil.

Transfer to the oven and leave to cook for 20–25 minutes, giving the mixture a stir with a spatula or wooden spoon halfway through cooking until the kale is nicely crisped. These are best served straight away, or within an hour of making.

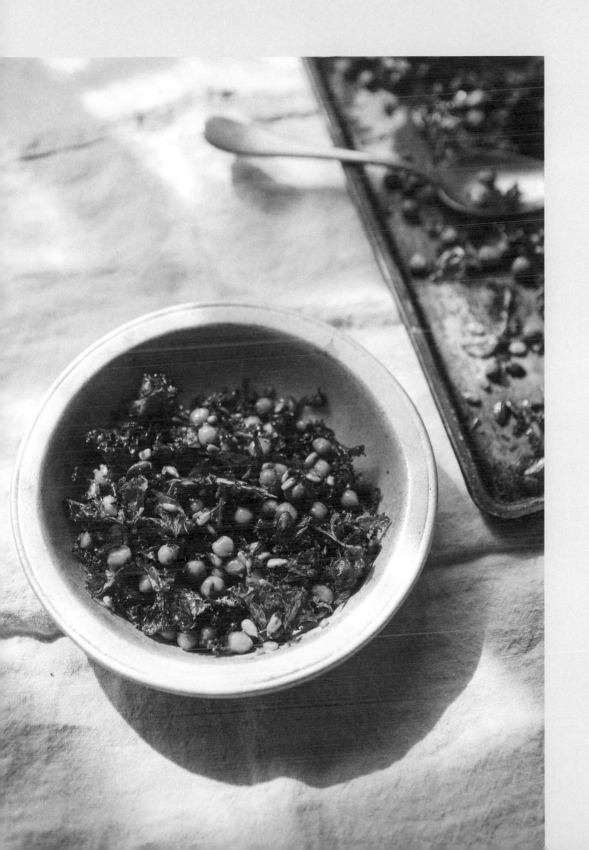

Dried Fruit Energy Balls

These fruit balls are perfect for when hunger strikes and you are in need of an energy boost. I love the combination of apricots and almonds because it makes these balls taste really creamy, and the cocoa adds a touch of decadence. Older kids will enjoy helping you roll these into balls. Reach for one of these whenever you need an instant pick-me-up.

Put the dates, almonds and dried apricots into a food processor and process until well combined. Add the coconut oil and cocoa powder and blitz again until the mixture has come together, gradually adding a little of the water if the mixture seems too dry.

Take tablespoonfuls of the mixture and roll together in your hands to form golf ball-sized balls. The mixture should make around 20. These are lovely as they are, but can also be rolled in more cocoa or desiccated coconut before serving for an added flourish.

Prep: 10 minutes
Makes 20

250 g/9 oz soft dates, pitted
100 g/3½ oz blanched whole
 almonds
100 g/3½ oz dried apricots
1 tbsp coconut oil
4 tbsp cocoa powder
1–2 tbsp water (optional)
unsweetened desiccated coconut
 or extra cocoa powder, for rolling
 (optional)

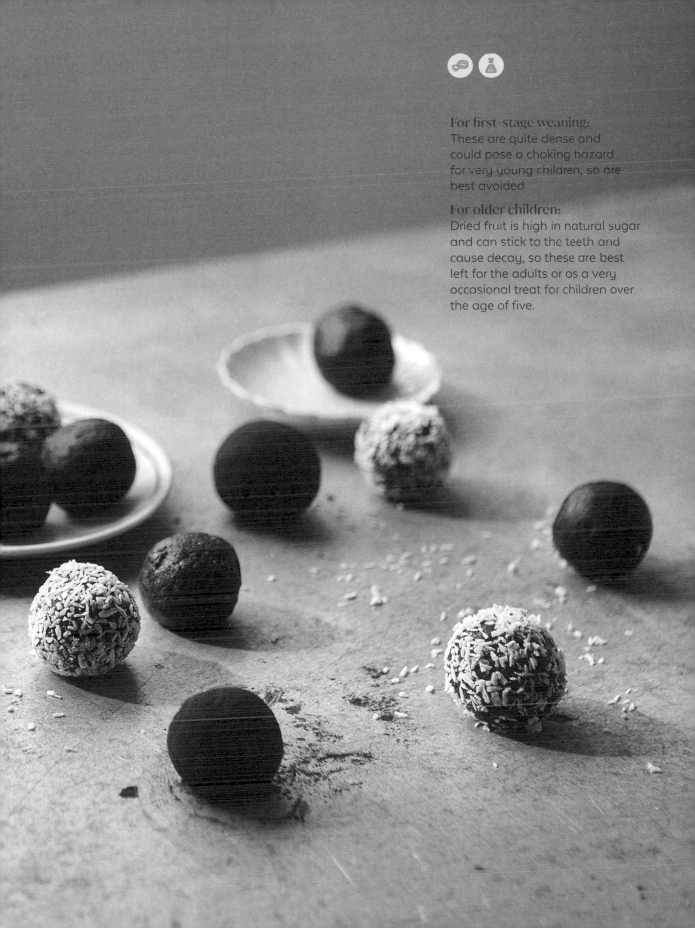

For first-stage weaning:
These are quite dense and could pose a choking hazard for very young children, so are best avoided

For older children:
Dried fruit is high in natural sugar and can stick to the teeth and cause decay, so these are best left for the adults or as a very occasional treat for children over the age of five.

Apple & Pear Crisps

Prep: 5 minutes
Cook: 1 hour 20 minutes, plus cooling
Serves 4–6

2 apples or 2 pears

For first-stage weaning:
Because these are fairly chewy, they are unsuitable for babies and children below 12 months.

For older children:
These are a great on-the-go snack for older children.

Like my Crunchy Chickpeas and Kale Crisps (see page 56), these dried apple and pear slices are a fantastic alternative to normal crisps. They are a doddle to make and contain no nasty added extras. Make these and store them in an airtight container, so you have easy snacks to hand. These are perfect for when you are out and about with the kids – I call them 'buggy snacks'. A handful of these will keep your toddler happy for ages.

Preheat the oven to 120°C/250°F/gas mark ½ and line 2–3 large baking sheets with greaseproof paper.

Slice the pears or apples as thinly as possible. For pears, it works best to slice from top to bottom, for apples, I like to slice across the core so that the pretty star shape is in the centre. The best way to do this is using a mandoline slicer or with the finest slicing blade on a food processor. If using a mandoline, you can leave the fruit whole to get nice cross-sections of apple or pear, but if using a food processor you will need to half the fruit so that it fits through the chute of the processor.

Lay the apple or pear slices flat on the prepared baking sheets, making sure that none of the slices overlaps, then transfer to the oven and bake for 40 minutes. Remove the baking sheets from the oven and turn all of the fruit slices over, then return to the oven and continue to cook for another 40 minutes. At this point, turn off the oven but leave the fruit on the baking sheets inside until cooled down to room temperature, when they should be crisp and delicious. These will keep in an airtight container for a few days.

Homemade Trail Mix

This is the ultimate powerhouse of treat snacks and a small handful is enough to put a smile back on the faces of the hungriest of kids. It takes seconds to put together and kids will enjoy helping. It is also very portable, so makes a great on-the-go snack option. This recipe is not set in stone – you may want to throw other things that you have in the cupboard like coconut flakes, sunflower seeds, or even plain popcorn.

Put all the ingredients into a large jar, seal and shake to combine. A handful of this makes the perfect mid-morning energy boost. Keep the jar sealed and it will keep for several weeks.

Prep: 2 minutes
Makes 250 g/9 oz

50 g/2 oz dried banana chips
50 g/2 oz blanched hazelnuts
50 g/2 oz whole almonds
50 g/2 oz dark chocolate chips
50 g/2 oz sultanas or raisins

For first-stage weaning:
This is not suitable for very young children, as whole nuts can present a choking hazard to under fives.

For older children:
As above, children below five years old should not be offered whole nuts because they are a potential choking hazard. For over fives, this makes a great occasional treat.

Three
Fun Food Games Your Kids Will Love

I know it can be messy, but letting your child play with food is great for their sensory development. It makes them more confident to try new foods because once they become familiar with them, they are more likely to accept and enjoy them. It's also a great, stealthy way to help them identify and name different foods, plus it really captures their attention, so you can have a few minutes of peace with a cup of tea! I know it might go over their (or your!) face and hair, but it's quickly washed off and most importantly they will love it. Here are some ideas for some fun food games:

Veggie Colour Match

What do you need?
· edible paints
· veggies and fruit

When doing this with the kids, I always put a big plastic sheet onto my table in an attempt to keep it clean, as this can get messy! Get hold of some child-friendly edible paint or make your own by combining cream cheese or vanilla yoghurt and edible food dye. Give your little one various chopped veggies and fruits, such as carrots (with orange paint), broccoli (with green paint), or strawberries (with red paint) and allow them to make prints on paper. This is a great activity to learn the names of the different colours and shapes, too.

Indoor 'Treasure' Sandbox

What do you need?
- a large container
- puffed rice cereal, dry pasta, dry rice or porridge oats (the sand!)
- measuring cups and other small containers
- small pieces of chopped soft fruit and veggies (the treasure!)

Chop colourful fruit and veggies into small pieces and hide them in your 'sand'. Encourage your child to dig around and explore to see what they can find. Puffed rice works best for younger children, but older toddlers can enjoy rummaging in other food items such as pasta and rice, and will find pouring their 'sand' using different measuring cups fun. My kids love playing together in this way.

Cereal Necklaces

What do you need?
- cereal snacks that are 'o' shaped or any other edible loops (try and use a sugar-free option if possible)
- piece of string (wool can become too wet)

Put your cereal snacks in a bowl and show your little one how to thread the cereal onto the string. This is ideal for children from around a year upwards and is great for their fine motor control. Don't worry if only half the cereal makes it onto the string. Once they have finished, tie a knot at the end and their necklace is ready. My girls love creating things like this – Valle is at that age where she is so proud of herself when she makes things!

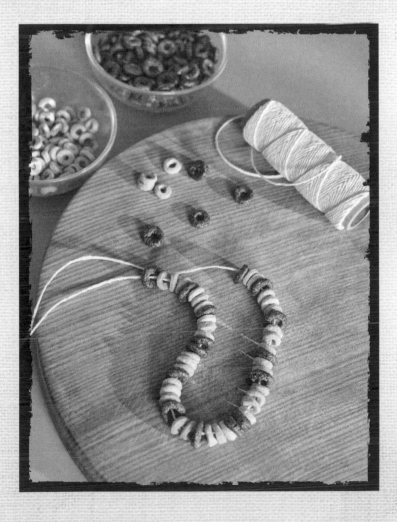

Try creating patterns in your necklaces by alternating different coloured cereals.

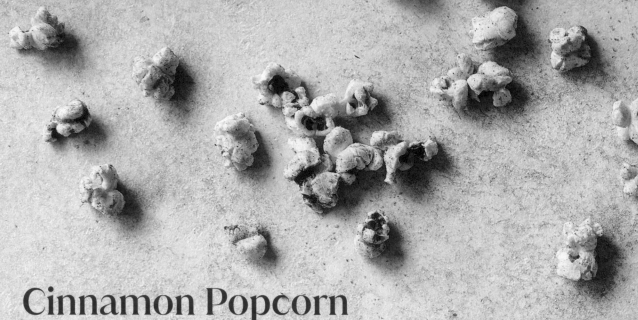

Cinnamon Popcorn

Freshly popped popcorn is great for movie nights at home. My kids love hearing the kernels pop and this recipe is a great twist on the classic. If you are stuck for original ideas, it is also a real hit at kids parties. The cinnamon gives the corn a really warming kick.

Put the sugar, butter and cinnamon in a small pan over a low heat and cook, stirring occasionally until the butter has melted and the sugar has dissolved.

Meanwhile, heat the oil in a separate pan. Once the oil is hot, add 3 or 4 popcorn kernels to the pan and swirl in the oil. Cover with a lid and leave until you hear the corn pop; this means the oil is at the right temperature. Add the rest of the popcorn kernels to the pan, cover with a lid and leave to cook until all the corn has popped, around 3 minutes.

Remove the pan from the heat and pour the butter and sugar mixture over the popcorn, then cover and shake the pan to ensure the popcorn is evenly coated. Serve warm.

For first-stage weaning:
Popcorn can present a choking hazard to very young children, so is best avoided. Instead, cut toast into soldiers and spread with cinnamon butter to involve them in the treat.

For older children:
Children age five and up can enjoy this as it is.

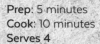

Prep: 5 minutes
Cook: 10 minutes
Serves 4

2 tbsp light soft brown sugar
15 g/½ oz unsalted butter
1 tsp ground cinnamon
1 tbsp sunflower oil
100 g/3½ oz popcorn kernels

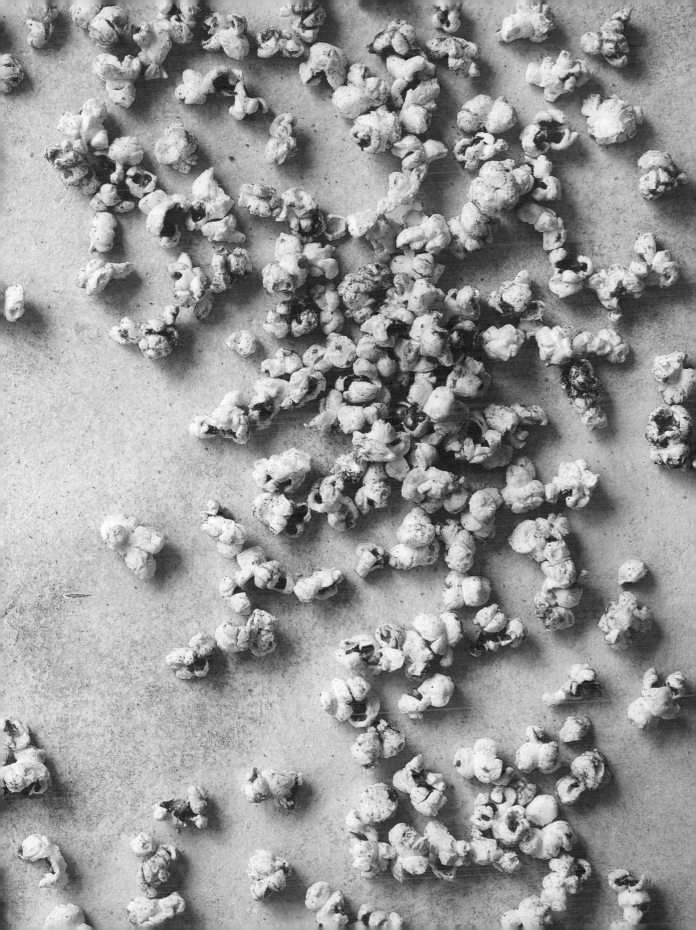

Oaty Apple & Pear Bars

Prep: 15 minutes
Cook: 20 minutes
Makes 12

1 apple, peeled, cored and grated
1 pear, peeled and grated
1 tsp ground cinnamon
225 ml/8 fl oz good-quality apple
   juice or coconut water
300 g/10½ oz porridge oats
100 g/3½ oz unsalted butter
100 ml/3½ fl oz clear honey or
   golden syrup

For first-stage weaning:
These contain honey so should
not be offered before your child is
12 months old. The soft texture of
these bars makes them good for
teething children.

For older children:
These are perfect lunchbox
snacks for older pre-schoolers
and school-age children.

These healthy bars are a fab source of slow-release
energy. They smell amazing when they are cooking
and are packed full of fibre. If children need to take
something to school with them for a morning snack or
in a lunch box (most schools have a 'no nut' policy due
to allergies), these are a great option. Because of their
soft texture, they are also ideal for younger children,
who will love holding and munching them.

Preheat the oven to 180°C/350°F/gas mark 4 and grease a
square 20-cm/8-inch baking pan with butter and line with
greaseproof paper.

Put the grated apple and pear in a large bowl along with
the cinnamon, apple juice or coconut water and half of
the porridge oats, then stir to combine and set aside for
20 minutes to soak.

Meanwhile, put the butter and honey in a large pan over a
medium heat. Once the butter has melted, remove the pan
from the heat and stir in the soaked oat, apple and pear
mixture, as well as the remaining dry oats.

Pour the mixture into the prepared baking pan and level out
the surface with a spatula, then transfer to the oven and leave
to cook for 20–25 minutes until golden and firm. Leave to cool
in the tin for 10–15 minutes, then use the greaseproof paper
to lift out of the tin. Slice into 12 equal-sized bars whilst still
warm. These can be eaten straight away, or left to cool to
room temperature. They will keep in an airtight container for
up to 5 days.

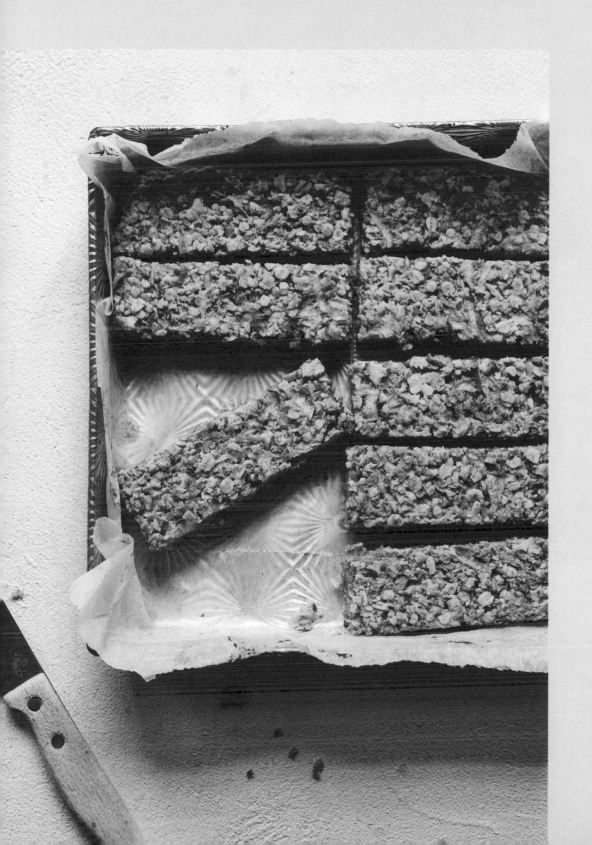

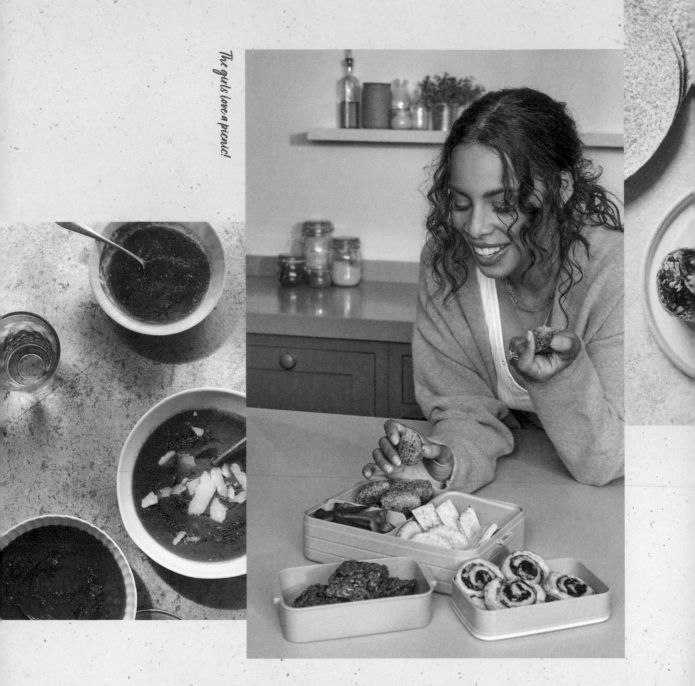

The girls love a picnic!

When you are home with the kids, it can be too easy to reach for the same lunch day after day, so hopefully my ideas will inspire you to shake things up a bit! From Rainbow Wraps (see page 92) and Tuna Melts (see page 79) to Sweet Potato Quesadillas (see page 87) and Halloumi (or Chicken) Fajitas (see page 72), everyone in the family will be able to get involved and will love these options. Many of these are so delicious you may also want to dish them up for dinner!

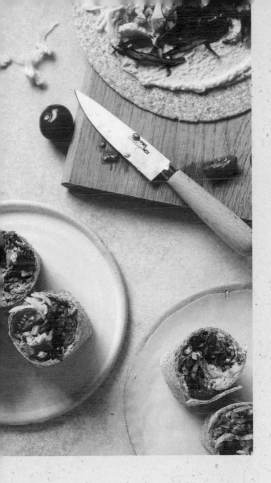

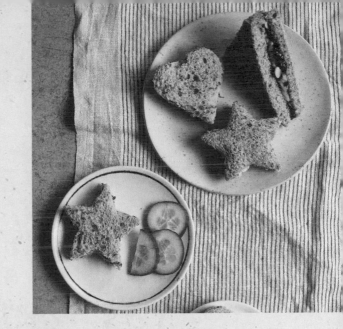

Lunch

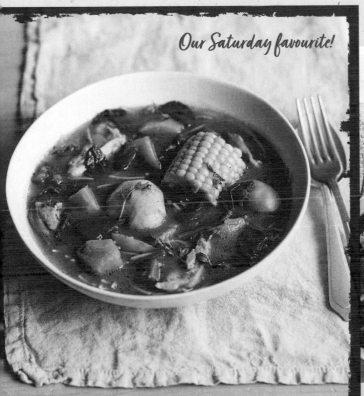

Our Saturday favourite!

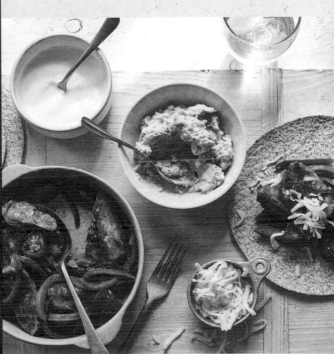

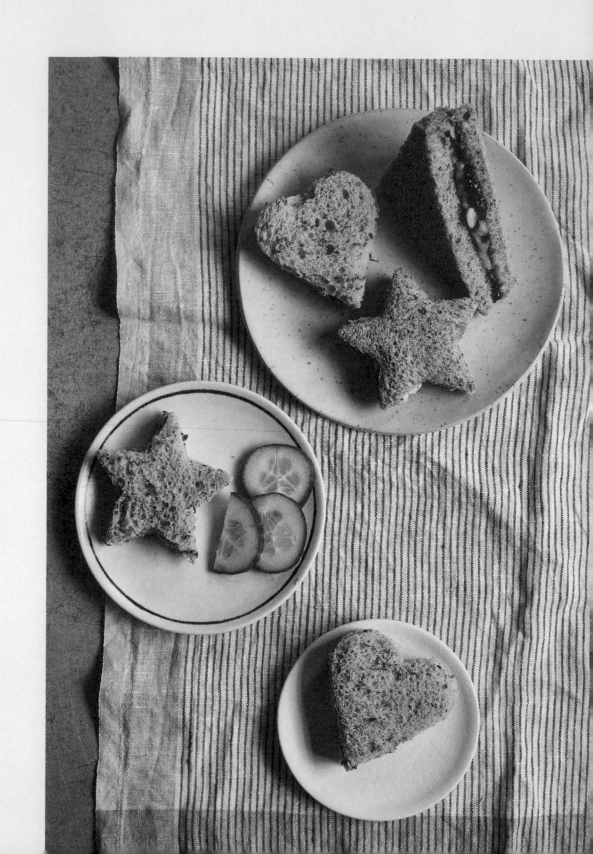

Fun Shaped Sandwiches

Making sandwiches for lunch boxes or lunch at home can become very boring (no wonder the kids get bored by them too!). This way of presenting them makes it all the more appealing and you can use whatever cookie cutter shapes you have to hand. Try to use wholemeal bread, so they are getting extra fibre. You can mix up the fillings depending on what your kids like, but I always try to get some fruit and veg in somewhere – even if it is just on the side as a little picnic-style lunch spread. Don't worry about the waste – the offcuts will make a tasty lunch for mum or dad!

Lay the bread on a board and butter the upward faces, slice off the crusts and cut the slices into 12 equal halves. Set aside while you prepare the sandwich fillings.

To make the tuna, mayonnaise and sweetcorn filling, fluke the tuna into a bowl, then add the sweetcorn and mayonnaise, stir to combine and season to taste.

To assemble the sandwiches, layer up the components for each sandwich type on 2 of the half-slices of bread, topping the tuna-mayonnaise with a layer of spinach leaves, and the ham and cream cheese with a layer of cucumber slices. (This should leave you with 6 topped pieces of bread, 2 of each filling.) Top the sandwiches with the remaining half slices of bread, then stamp or cut the sandwiches into your desired shapes. I have suggested triangles for the tuna mayo, stars for the cream cheese and ham, and hearts for the banana and jam, but use whatever shape cutters you have to hand.

Prep: 15 minutes
Makes 12 small sandwiches

6 large slices wholemeal bread
butter, for spreading

For the tuna mayo & sweetcorn triangles
1 x 160 g/5¾ oz can tuna in spring water, drained
1 x 200 g/7 oz can sweetcorn, drained
2 tbsp mayonnaise
20 g/¾ oz spinach leaves
sea salt and freshly ground black pepper

For the cream cheese, ham & cucumber stars
2 tbsp cream cheese
4 slices good-quality sliced ham
70 g/2½ oz cucumber, thinly sliced

For the mashed banana and raspberry jam hearts
2 ripe bananas, peeled and mashed until smooth
2 tbsp strawberry jam

For first-stage weaning:
Serve weaning babies the crusts from the bread spread with cream cheese, along with batons of cucumber and some mashed banana.

For older children:
Children will love with these mini sandwiches. Always check for any allergies if serving children who are not your own.

Halloumi (or Chicken) Fajitas

Prep: 10 minutes
Cook: 10 minutes
Serves 4

350 g/12 oz halloumi or chicken breast
1 tsp smoked paprika or fajita seasoning
1 tbsp olive oil, plus extra, for drizzling
2 peppers (red, orange or green), deseeded and sliced
1 small red onion, halved and sliced
180 g/6 oz cherry tomatoes, halved
1-2 ripe avocados
8 small wholemeal tortillas
100 g/3½ oz natural yoghurt
80 g/3 oz Cheddar cheese, grated
sliced red chillies (optional)
sea salt and freshly ground black pepper

For first-stage weaning:
Cook some of the vegetables without any seasoning, then blitz to a purée and serve with some unseasoned mashed avocado and tortillas cut into strips.

For older children:
Older children may prefer their halloumi or chicken without any spice. Omit the seasoning when mashing the avocado and serve the chillies on the side, so that there are no unwanted surprises for young palates.

Halloumi is a great alternative to chicken in fajitas. I like to cut it into strips rather than chunks, which gives it a meatier texture. If you're not a fan of halloumi, you can use chicken here if you would rather – I've given instructions for both in the method. Mix in whatever veg you have in the fridge (those multi packs of peppers are ideal here.) Try to use cherry tomatoes on the vine, as the flavour is sweeter.

If using halloumi, cut the block into 5 mm/¼ inch slices, then cut each slice in half to make long strips. If using chicken, cut the chicken breast into strips. Add the halloumi or chicken to a bowl along with the smoked paprika or fajita seasoning and a drizzle of olive oil, and toss so that everything is coated in the spices.

Heat the oil in a wok or large frying pan over a medium heat. Add the halloumi or chicken and cook, stirring, for 5 minutes until golden. Tip the halloumi or chicken into a bowl and set aside, then return the pan to heat and add the sliced peppers, red onion and cherry tomatoes, and cook, stirring occasionally, for 5 minutes until the vegetables are tender and slightly charred. Return the halloumi or chicken to the pan and stir briefly to combine with the vegetables, then remove the pan from the heat.

While the vegetables are cooking, half the avocados and remove the stones, then scoop the flesh into a bowl, season with salt and pepper, and mash with a fork until smooth.

Warm the tortillas briefly in a separate pan or in the toaster or microwave, then bring to the table along with bowls of the cooked chicken and vegetables, mashed avocado, natural yoghurt, grated cheese and sliced chillies, if using. Allow everyone to top the tortillas with their choice of fillings, then wrap up and enjoy.

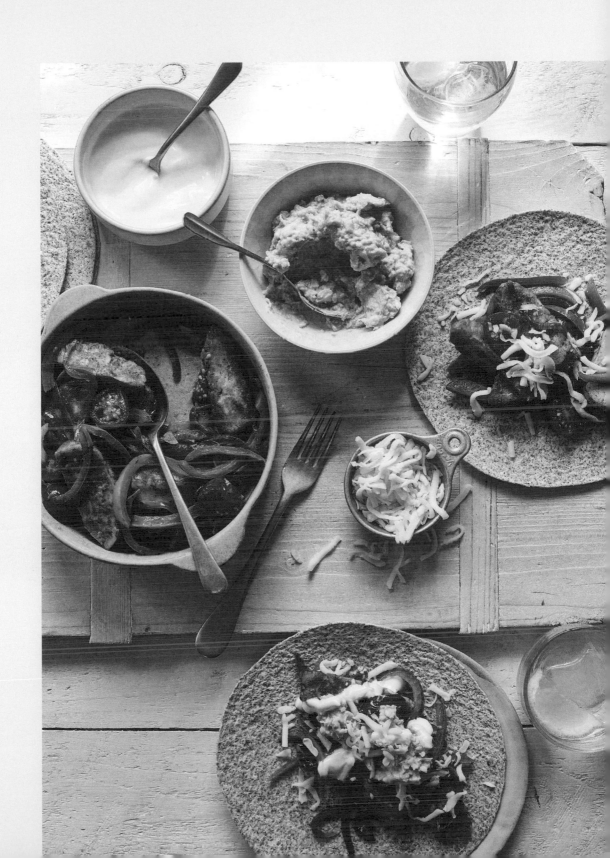

This traditional Caribbean soup is Marvin's dad's speciality. He used to make it for us every Saturday and now I do the same, so it feels like a real ritual. It is packed with flavour and is really filling. I have simplified it a little here as you would normally brine the chicken, but instead I have marinated it quickly with lemon, sea salt and pepper to save time. The result is still delicious!

For first-stage weaning:
This soup isn't suitable for weaning children, though you could serve them some of the chopped peppers and carrot and a portion of plain noodles so that they feel like they are part of the meal.

For older children:
This soup has a kick that children may find challenging. You could make a plainer broth by omitting the spice and chilli, and cook the dumplings and veg in the same way so that they feel like they're eating the same meal as the adults at the table.

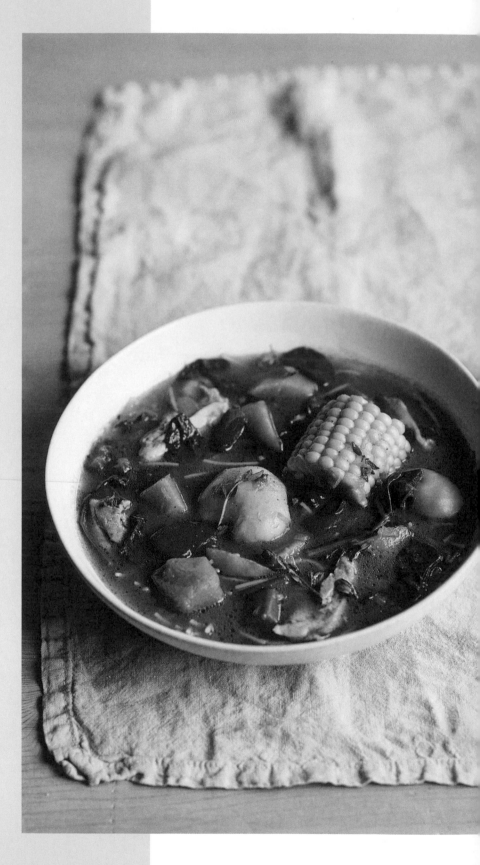

Lunch

Pops' Saturday Soup

Remove the skin from the chicken thighs and discard, then, using a heavy knife, cut each thigh in half through the bone – you may need to give the blade of the knife a gentle whack with a rolling pin to help with this. Put the chicken in a bowl, season with salt and pepper and pour over the lemon juice, then cover and leave in the fridge to marinate while you make the dumplings.

To make the dumplings, put the flour and a pinch of salt in a bowl and pour over most of the water, bringing the mixture together with your hands until it forms a dough and adding a little more if necessary. Put in the fridge for 15 minutes to firm up while you start the base for the soup.

Heat the olive oil in a large pan over a medium heat, then add the onion and cook, stirring, for 10 minutes until soft and golden. Add the carrot, pepper, garlic and bay leaves to the pan, stir to combine with the onions, then cover with a lid and leave to cook for 2 minutes. Season with salt and pepper, stir through the jerk seasoning, then replace the lid and cook for a further 2 minutes.

Meanwhile, remove the dough for the dumplings from the fridge and cut into quarters, then cut each quarter into 3. Roll each piece of dough into a ball with your hands, so that you have 12 equal-sized dumplings. Set aside while you continue to build the soup.

Remove the lid from the pan and pour in the stock, then add the potatoes and butternut squash. Bring the mixture to the boil, then reduce to a simmer and cook for 15 minutes, stirring occasionally. Add the chicken, dumplings, spinach and thyme sprigs to the pan and stir to combine, bring the mixture back to a simmer, then place the scotch bonnet on top of the soup and leave to cook for a final 15 minutes.

While the soup is cooking, cook the noodles according to packet instructions, then divide between 4 serving bowls. Pick out the chilli, bay leaves and thyme sprigs, then ladle the soup into the bowls, ensuring that everyone gets a good mix of chicken, veg and dumplings. Serve hot.

Prep: 20 minutes, plus resting
Cook: 45 minutes
Serves 4

4 skin-on, bone-in chicken thighs (approx. 450 g/1 lb)
juice of 1 lemon
250 g/9 oz plain flour
150 ml/5 fl oz water
2 tbsp olive oil
1 large onion, roughly chopped
1 carrot, peeled and cut into 1 cm/ ½ in pieces
1 red pepper, deseeded and sliced
5 garlic cloves, crushed
2 bay leaves
2 tsp jerk seasoning
1.4 litres/2½ pints chicken stock
700 g/1 lb 9 oz white potatoes, peeled and cut into 2 cm/¾ in chunks
450 g/1 lb butternut squash or pumpkin, peeled, deseeded and cut into bite-sized chunks
40 g/1½ oz spinach leaves
6 sprigs thyme
1 scotch bonnet chilli
100 g/3½ oz vermicelli noodles
sea salt and freshly ground black pepper

Simple Playdate Recipes

My kids love having their friends over to play and I always try to include food on playdates that I know my own kids and their guests will enjoy. These recipes hit the sweet spot of being simple, healthy and always going down well.

Traffic Light Pasta

Prep: 5 minutes
Cook: 15 minutes
Serves 4

350 g/12 oz wholemeal penne pasta or dried coloured pasta
1 tbsp olive oil
1 onion, halved and finely sliced
1 garlic clove, crushed
½ orange pepper, deseeded and chopped into 1 cm/½ in pieces
100 g/3½ oz frozen peas
1 x 400 g/14 oz can chopped tomatoes
240 g/9 oz mozzarella
sea salt and freshly ground black pepper

For first-stage weaning:
Omit the seasoning and only add half the pasta to the sauce, then blitz the sauce, pasta and all, to a purée. Serve the purée with the reserved pasta alongside so that children can grab pieces to chew, which helps develop their fine-motor skills.

For older children:
Omit the seasoning and pass around to the adults only when serving the meal.

This is a really fun and colourful lunch option that will appeal to little and big kids alike with its traffic light of green peas, orange peppers and red tomatoes. I try to stick to wholemeal pasta where possible as it contains more fibre. You can also try fun-coloured pasta, such as lentil and beetroot which the kids love, and I often switch it up to include different shapes. The girls love farfalle - the little bows - but I will often have a few different styles in my cupboard.

Bring a large pan of water to the boil over a medium heat. Add the pasta and a pinch of salt, then reduce the heat to a simmer and cook, according to packet instructions until tender.

Meanwhile, heat the olive oil in a large frying pan over a medium heat. Add the onion, garlic and pepper and cook, stirring continuously, for 5 minutes until soft. Tip in the chopped tomatoes, then refill the can with water and tip that in, too. Give the mixture a stir, bring back to a simmer and leave to cook, stirring occasionally, for 5 minutes.

Drain the pasta, reserving a mug of the pasta water. Add the pasta, pasta water and peas to the pan with the tomato mixture and stir until everything is well combined and the pasta is coated with the sauce. Season to taste, then tear over the mozzarella, spoon into serving bowls and serve.

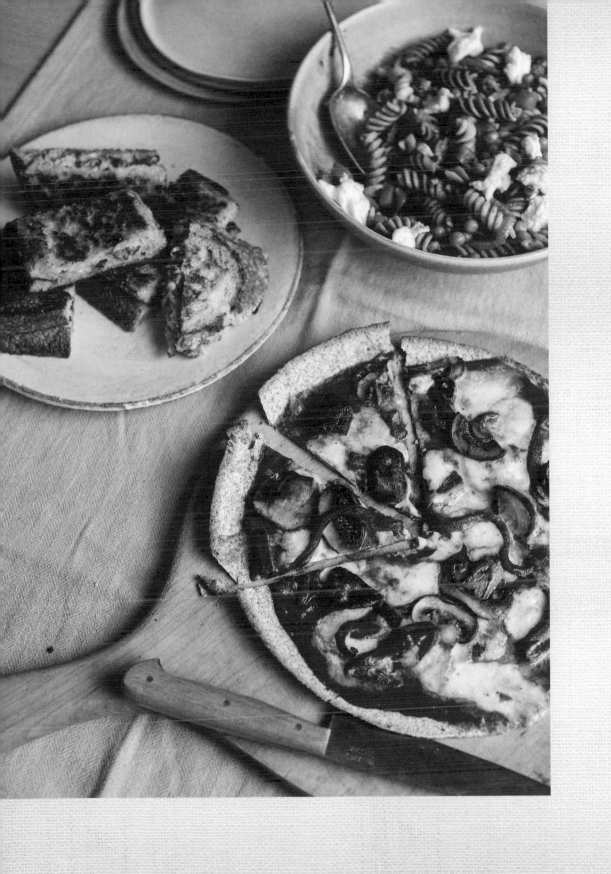

Tortilla Pizzas

My kids love these and making them is a great playdate activity – who doesn't want help in the kitchen and to keep the kids entertained at the same time? This also makes a great last-minute go-to – you can just see what toppings you have in the fridge. The tomato sauce recipe makes more than you will need for these pizzas, but it keeps well in the fridge or freezer and can be used to dress pasta for an easy-win dinner later in the week. The ingredients for each topping makes enough for 1 pizza, so you can make four of one type or mix and match according to your preference.

Prep: 20 minutes
Cook: 3–5 minutes
Serves 4

1 x 430 g/15 oz jar passata
handful of basil leaves
½ garlic clove, crushed
4 large wholemeal tortilla wraps

For the Margarita topping:
¼ ball mozzarella
handful of basil leaves

For the ham & pineapple topping:
40 g/1½ oz good-quality sliced ham, torn into strips
100 g/3½ oz canned pineapple, cut into bite-sized chunks
¼ ball mozzarella

For the roasted veggie topping:
50 g/2 oz chestnut mushrooms, finely sliced
¼ red pepper, deseeded and sliced
65 g/2½ oz courgette, coarsely grated
¼ ball mozzarella

Optional extras:
handful of rocket
good grating of Parmesan
sea salt and freshly ground black pepper
spinach and avocado salad, to serve

For first-stage weaning:
Blitz up some of the roasted veg with the tomato sauce to make a thick purée.

For older children:
Serve the pizza as it is, but leave off the rocket and extra Parmesan.

If you are making the roasted veggie pizza, preheat the oven to 200°C/400°F/gas mark 6 and line a baking sheets with foil. Spread the sliced mushrooms and peppers out on the prepared baking sheet and transfer to the oven for 15 minutes until tender. Remove from the oven and increase the temperature to 220°C/425°F/gas mark 7.

For all other pizzas, simply preheat the oven to 220°C/425°F/gas mark 7.

To make the tomato sauce, put the passata, garlic and basil leaves into a blender and pulse until smooth and well combined.

Lay the tortillas flat on the remaining 2 baking sheets and spread each with 1 tablespoon of the tomato sauce, leaving a 5 mm/¼ inch border around the edges. Layer the pizzas with your chosen toppings and finish by tearing the mozzarella over the top of each.

Bake in the oven for 2–3 minutes until golden and bubbling. Top the pizzas with a handful of rocket leaves and a sprinkling of Parmesan, if using. Slice and serve with a spinach and avocado salad alongside.

Tuna Melts

I find the combination of tuna and hot cheese irresistible. Ideally, you need good bakery bread because it is a bit thicker, so toasts really well. Sometimes thinner, pre-sliced bread from supermarkets burns quite easily. If you are using this type of bread, just keep it on a lower heat. My kids love this recipe too. Tuna is a great source of protein and contains all the important amino acids needed for growth.

Put a heavy-based frying pan over a medium heat to warm up while you prepare the sandwiches.

Lay the bread on a board and butter the upward faces. Flake the tuna into a bowl, then add the spring onions, mayonnaise, grated Cheddar and chopped spinach, and stir until well combined.

Flip over 3 pieces of the bread so that the buttered sides are facing down, then spread each of these with a third of the tuna mixture. Close the sandwiches with another slice of bread, this time with the butter facing up, so that the buttered sides of each piece of bread are on the outside of the sandwiches.

Transfer the assembled sandwiches to the hot pan (depending on the size of your pan, you may need to do this in batches), then reduce the heat to low. Leave to cook for 2–3 minutes until crisp and golden on the underside, then flip the sandwiches and cook for another 2–3 minutes. To get the sandwiches extra crisp, I like to rest a heavy-based pan on them to press them down while cooking.

Transfer the toasties to a board and slice into halves or quarters, then serve with salad, and batons of carrot and cucumber on the side and tomato ketchup for dipping.

Prep: 5 minutes
Cook: 5 minutes
Serves 4

6 thick slices wholemeal or sourdough bread
butter, for spreading
1 x 160 g/5¾ oz can tuna in spring water, drained
3 spring onions, finely sliced
3 tbsp mayonnaise
50 g/2 oz Cheddar cheese, grated
20 g/¾ oz spinach leaves, finely chopped
tomato ketchup, salad, carrot and cucumber sticks, to serve

For first-stage weaning:
Blitz up the tuna, Cheddar and spinach, spread onto toast and cut into soldiers to serve.

For older children:
Children with sensitive palates may not like the spring onions, so leave those out if your children aren't keen. Otherwise the sandwiches can be enjoyed as they are.

Roasted Veggie & Chickpea Quinoa Salad

Prep: 10 minutes
Cook: 40 minutes
Serves 4

1 courgette, cut into 2 cm/¾ in chunks
1 aubergine, cut into 2 cm/¾ in chunks
½ red pepper, deseeded and cut into 2 cm/¾ in chunks
1 x 400 g/14 oz can chickpeas, drained
2 tbsp olive oil
150 g/5 oz quinoa or couscous
50 g/2 oz spinach leaves, roughly chopped
zest and juice of 1 lemon
80 g/3 oz mozzarella, torn
30 g/1 oz shelled pistachios, roughly chopped
sea salt and freshly ground black pepper

For first-stage weaning:
Roast a small portion of the veg without seasoning, then serve with some mashed up or puréed chickpeas and couscous or quinoa.

For older children:
Depending on your children's tastes, you may want to portion out some of the quinoa and roasted veg before adding the spinach and pistachios.

Roasting veg is a great way to add depth of flavour and is easy to prepare in advance. You can make a big batch and use any extra to add to soups, salads, or blitz up with a tin of tomatoes to make a pasta sauce. I have included my favourite veg for this recipe, but if you have other veggies that need to be used up in the fridge, this is a great way to use them.

Preheat the oven to 200°C/400°F/gas mark 6 and line a roasting tin with foil.

Put the courgette, aubergine, red pepper and chickpeas in the roasting tin and drizzle over the olive oil. Season with salt and pepper, then give the tin a shake to ensure the veg are evenly coated in the oil. Transfer to the oven for 30–40 minutes until the veg are tender and golden.

While the vegetables are in the oven, cook the quinoa or couscous according to packet instructions, then tip into a large serving bowl and set aside until needed.

Once the veg are cooked, tip them into the bowl with the quinoa or couscous, then add the lemon zest and juice, spinach, mozzarella and chopped pistachios. Toss everything until really well combined, then season to taste and serve.

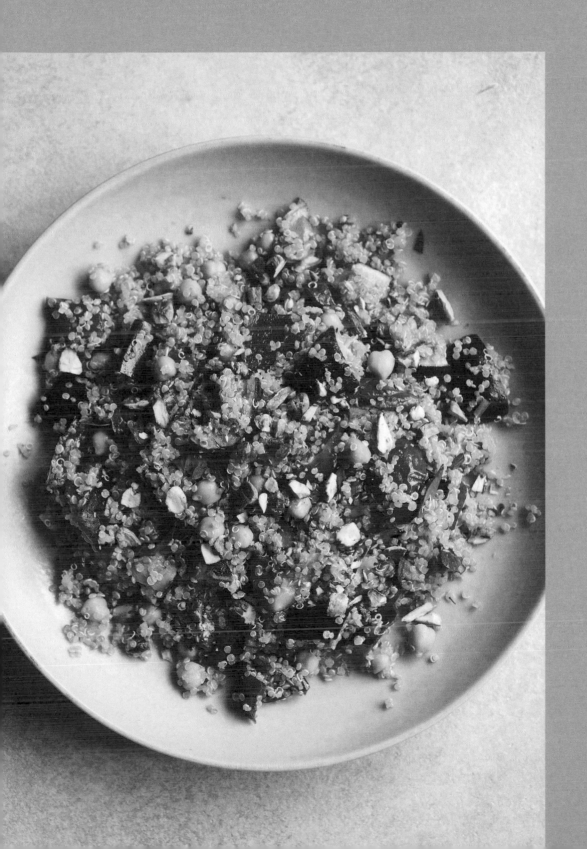

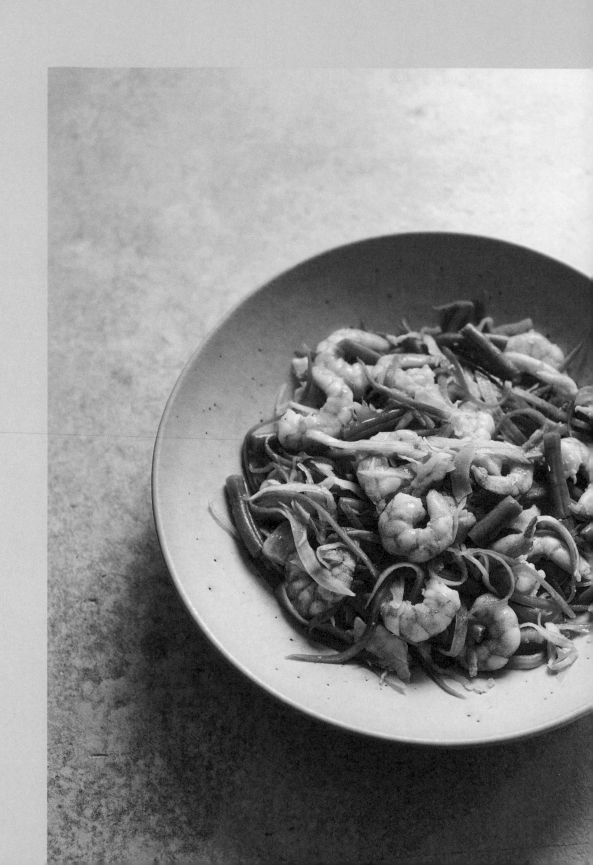

Asian Prawn Salad

We adore Asian food and this is one of my go-to salad recipes. It has a mouthwatering sweet-and-savoury kick and an irresistible crunchy texture. Top this with as much or as little tangy dressing as you wish. This is great for a summer supper, plus lunch the next day if you have leftovers. The sauce is particularly moreish and it is so easy to eat the whole bowl without even realising. Preparing the veg is the work of moments if you have a food processor.

To make the dressing, put the lime juice, tamarind paste, fish sauce, soy sauce, caster sugar and garlic in a small bowl and stir to combine. Slowly whisk in the oil until everything has come together to a smooth dressing. Set aside while you prepare the salad.

Bring a small pan of water to the boil over a medium heat, then add the chopped green beans and cook for 5 minutes until just tender but still retaining some bite. Drain and transfer to a large bowl, along with the prepared carrots and cabbage. Pour the dressing over the salad and toss everything to combine. Set aside while you cook the prawns.

Heat the sesame oil in a frying pan over a medium heat. Add the prawns to the pan and cook, stirring continuously, for 5 minutes until pink on the outside and cooked through. Tip the prawns into the bowl with the salad and give everything a final toss to combine all of the elements. Divide the salad between serving plates and serve.

Prep: 10 minutes
Cook: 5 minutes
Serves 4

100 g/3½ oz green beans, trimmed and cut into thirds
2 carrots, peeled and grated or finely sliced
300 g/10½ oz white cabbage, shredded or finely chopped
1 tsp sesame oil
250 g/9 oz raw king prawns

For the dressing:
juice of 3 large limes
6 tbsp tamarind paste
3 tbsp fish sauce
3 tbsp reduced-salt soy sauce
2 tbsp caster sugar
1 garlic clove, finely grated
2 tbsp sesame oil

For first-stage weaning:
Shellfish, though an allergen, can be introduced from 6 months, just ensure that the prawns are thoroughly cooked to avoid risk of food poisoning. Cook some sliced carrots with the green beans, then blitz to a purée and serve alongside the prawns.

For older children:
Children may find the dressing a little punchy for their tastes, so serve the salad undressed, allowing everyone to add as much or as little dressing as they like.

Jacket Potatoes –Three Ways

Prep: 20 minutes
Cook: 1 hour
Serves 4

4 medium baking potatoes
2 tbsp olive oil
sea salt
butter, to serve
4 Cos lettuce leaves, shredded
handful of cherry tomatoes, halved

For the cheese, bean & bacon filling:
1 x 400 g/14 oz can baked beans
4 spring onions, finely sliced
4 rashers smoked streaky bacon,
   roughly chopped
½ tsp smoked paprika
85 g/3 oz Cheddar cheese, grated

For the hummus & mackerel filling:
85 g/3 oz hummus
140 g/5 oz smoked mackerel fillet,
   skin removed and flesh flaked

You can never go wrong with a humble spud. If I'm in a rush, I'll sometimes start these in the microwave for a few minutes before putting them in the oven. I've included some of my favourite toppings here – the kids' favourite is cheese, beans and bacon, but they also love hummus and smoked mackerel. Each of the filling recipes makes enough for all 4 potatoes, so scale them down if you want to mix and match.

Preheat the oven to 180°C/350°F/gas mark 4 and line a baking sheet with foil.

Prick the potatoes with a fork all over, then place on the baking sheet and drizzle with the olive oil. Scatter over some sea salt, then rub the salt and oil into the skin of the potatoes, ensuring they are evenly covered. Transfer to the oven and bake for 1 hour until the potatoes are crisp and golden on the outside and soft and fluffy on the inside.

Cut open the potatoes and spread with butter, then add your choice of fillings and serve with the lettuce and tomatoes on the side.

FOR THE CHEESE, BEAN AND BACON FILLING:
Put the beans in a small pan over a medium heat. Bring just to the boil, then reduce the heat to a simmer and add the spring onions, bacon and paprika. Cook, stirring occasionally, for 5 minutes until the spring onions are soft and the bacon is crisp. Spoon into the potatoes and scatter over the grated cheese to serve.

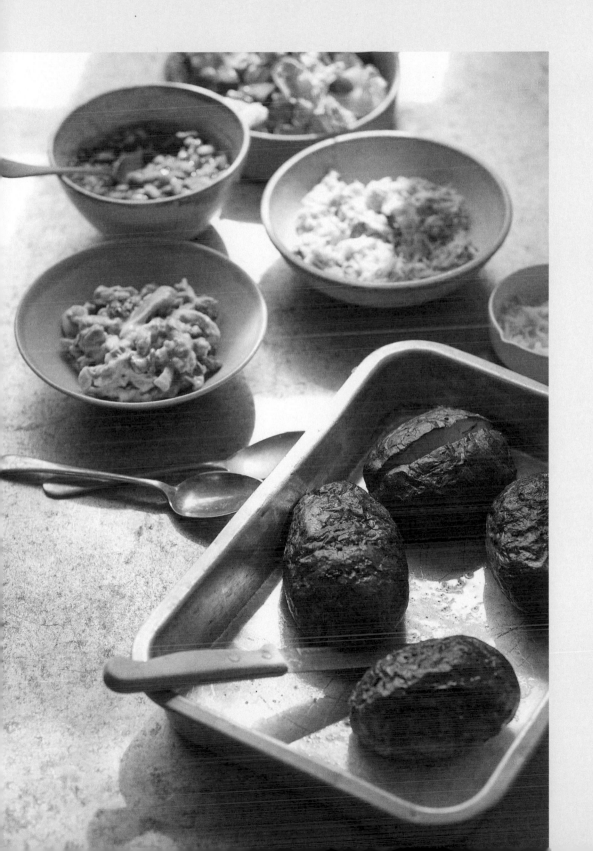

For the coronation chicken filling:
1 x 200 g/7 oz skinless, boneless
  chicken breast
1 tbsp olive oil
3 tbsp mayonnaise
1 tsp mild curry powder
1 heaped tbsp mango chutney
1 heaped tbsp sultanas or raisins
2 tbsp Greek yoghurt

For first-stage weaning:

Scoop out some of the insides of
the potato and serve mashed,
with grated cheese and reduced-
salt-and-sugar baked beans.

For older children:

Older children will enjoy these as
they are. Just leave the salt off
their potatoes before baking and
try and use a reduced-salt-and-
sugar variety of baked beans.

FOR THE CORONATION CHICKEN FILLING:

Lay the chicken breast flat on a chopping board and
cover with a sheet of greaseproof paper. Using a rolling pin
or heavy-based pan, bash the chicken breast to flatten to
a thickness of 1 cm/½ inch. Heat the oil in a frying pan over
a medium heat, then add the chicken breast and cook for
2–3 minutes on each side until cooked through. Set aside to
cool, while you make the coronation dressing.

Put the mayonnaise, curry powder, mango chutney, sultanas
or raisins and Greek yoghurt in a bowl and stir to combine.
Shred the cooled chicken and stir through the sauce, then
spoon the mixture into the jacket potatoes and serve.

FOR THE HUMMUS AND MACKEREL FILLING:

Spoon the hummus into the potatoes and top with the
shredded smoked mackerel. Serve.

That's a Wrap – Picnic & on-the-Move Food

Are you looking for food inspiration for days out? I love preparing picnic food with the girls and for days like schools sports days, where we spend time with other families outside. Here are some ideas for inspiration.

Sweet Potato Quesadillas

This is my sweeter twist on the traditional Mexican dish. I love using sweet potatoes because they add colour and flavour and, despite their name, they also contain more vitamins, minerals, and fibre than white potatoes. Add chilli sauce for an extra kick.

Pile the grated sweet potato onto the centre of a clean tea towel, then bring up the sides to enclose. Working over a sink or large bowl, twist the base of the tea towel as tightly as you can to remove any excess water. Tip the sweet potato into a large bowl and add the spring onions, cheese and chives. If you are making this for children and adults, you may want to divide the mixture at this point and season the adult portion only.

Put a large frying pan over a medium heat and, once hot, lay one of the tortilla wraps in the pan. Spoon over half of the filling mixture, pressing it down so it reaches almost to the edges of the wrap, then top with another wrap. Cook for 2–3 minutes until the bottom wrap is crisp and golden, then flip the quesadilla in the pan and cook for another 2–3 minutes until crisp on the outside and tender and melty on the inside. Transfer the quesadilla to a board while you repeat the process with the remaining wraps and filling.

Once both quesadillas are cooked, slice them into wedges and arrange on serving plates. Mix the yoghurt with the chilli sauce, if using, and serve alongside for dipping.

Prep: 5 minutes
Cook: 6 minutes
Serves 4

1 sweet potato, peeled and coarsely grated
4 spring onions, finely sliced
75 g/3 oz Cheddar cheese, grated
4 large wholemeal tortilla wraps
small bunch chives, snipped
4 tbsp natural yoghurt
2 tsp chilli sauce (optional)
sea salt and freshly ground black pepper

For first-stage weaning:
Chop some of the sweet potato into cubes, then microwave or boil for 5 minutes until tender. Blitz or mash the cooked sweet potato until smooth, then stir through some yoghurt and grated cheese.

For older children:
Serve older children the quesadillas as they are, but with natural yoghurt alongside and omitting the seasoning from the filling mixture.

Cheese & Marmite Pinwheels

Prep: 10-15 minutes
Cook: 15 minutes
Makes 20

375 g/13 oz ready-rolled puff pastry
1½ tbsp Marmite or other yeast
    extract
75 g/3 oz Cheddar cheese, grated

For first-stage weaning:
Omit the Marmite, but make the
pinwheels in the same way.

For older children:
Older children can enjoy these
as they are.

These are super-easy to make and can be prepared
in advance up to the baking stage, then chilled for
convenience, in which case you will need to bake for
15-20 minutes. Mix up the cheese you use for variety
– Cheddar is a classic, but you can use Red Leicester
or even crumbled feta cheese. We like a mature
cheddar in ours.

Preheat the oven to 200°C/400°F/gas mark 6 and line
a large baking sheet with greaseproof paper.

Unroll the puff pastry on its lining paper on the kitchen
counter with the longest side facing towards you. Use the
back of a spoon to spread the Marmite over the surface,
leaving a thin border around the edge of the pastry, then
scatter over the grated cheese.

Starting with one of the long edges and rolling away from
you, roll the pastry as tightly as possible, peeling away the
lining paper as you do so until you are left with a tightly rolled
sausage shape.

Slice the rolled dough into 2 cm/¾ inch rounds (you should
get about 20) and lay them flat on the prepared baking
sheet, leaving space between each to allow the pinwheels
to spread during cooking. Transfer to the oven and cook for
15-18 minutes until puffed up, crisp and golden. Transfer to a
wire rack and leave to cool. These will keep for a few days in
an airtight container.

If you want to make these ahead, simply freeze the sliced
pinwheels before baking, then bake directly from the freezer,
increasing the cooking time to 25 minutes.

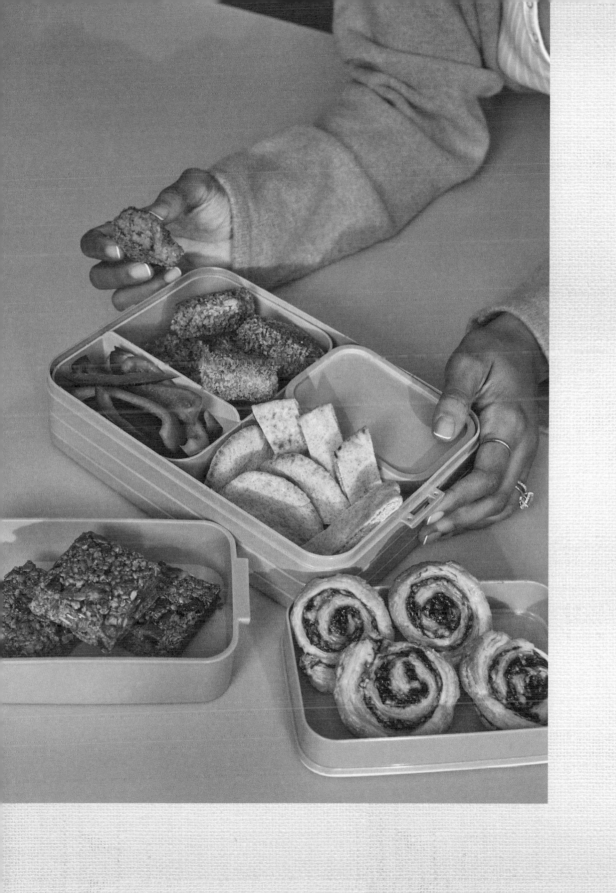

Falafel – Three Ways

Prep: 20 minutes
Cook: 10 minutes
Makes about 14

For the falafel base:
½ onion, roughly chopped (use red
   onion if making the beetroot falafel)
1 garlic clove, crushed
1 x 400 g/9 oz can chickpeas,
   drained
4 sprigs parsley, leaves picked (use
   mint if you are making the spinach
   and pea falafel)
3 heaped tbsp plain flour
½ tsp ground cumin
½ tsp ground coriander
150 g/5½ oz breadcrumbs
1 large egg
sea salt and freshly ground black
   pepper
vegetable oil, for frying

**For the chickpea & sweet potato
   falafel:**
1 sweet potato (approx. 300 g/
   10½ oz), baked until soft,
   then cooled

For the beetroot falafel:
140 g/5 oz cooked beetroot, roughly
   chopped

For the spinach and pea falafel:
100 g/3½ oz frozen peas, defrosted
50 g/1¾ oz fresh spinach leaves,
   rinsed

Falafel make such a wholesome and satisfying lunch choice. These recipes all have the same base, but I've mixed up the veg to give you three colourful options. The base recipe makes enough mixture for just one of the flavours, so pick which type of falafel you would like to make before you start, or scale up the falafel base recipe and make all three. They keep really well in the freezer if you make more than you need. This is the perfect meal for veggie lovers and veggie dodgers alike, as they are so colourful and appealing that kids will forget to ask what's in them! These can be eaten as they are, with hummus, or served with salad in a wrap.

Put the onion or red onion and garlic into the bowl of a food processor and blitz until smooth. Add the drained chickpeas and parsley or mint leaves, as well as the supplementary veg, depending on which flavour of falafel you have decided on and blitz the mixture again until smooth and well combined.

Tip the mixture into a large bowl and add the flour, ground cumin, ground coriander, 2 tablespoons of the breadcrumbs and a generous grinding of salt and pepper. Mix well to combine.

Set 2 shallow bowls next to each other on the work surface. Crack the egg into the first bowl and beat to combine, then add the remaining breadcrumbs to the second bowl.

Pour the vegetable oil into a large pan to a depth of 4 cm/1½ inches and place over a medium heat. Heat the oil to 180°C/350°F, using a cooking thermometer to monitor the temperature, or until a little of the mixture starts to bubble and fry when added to the pan.

While the oil is coming up to temperature, divide the falafel mixture into 14 equal-sized pieces and roll into balls with your hands. Press down on each ball slightly to create a disc shape, then dip each first into the egg and then into the breadcrumbs to coat.

Once the oil is at temperature, carefully add half of the falafel to the pan and fry in the oil for 5 minutes, turning halfway through cooking until crisp and golden. Use a slotted spoon to transfer the cooked falafel to a plate lined with kitchen paper to soak up any excess oil while you repeat the process with the remaining falafel.

The falafel can be served warm or cooled to room temperature. Serve with your choice of salad, hummus, pitta breads or wraps and with chilli sauce alongside.

For first-stage weaning:

Omit the seasoning from the falafel mixture and reduce the spicing by half for very young children. If your children prefer purées to solids, blitz some of the chickpeas with a little yoghurt and some of the veg from each type of falafel.

For older children:

Older children will enjoy these as they are, though you may want to reduce the seasoning or, better yet, portion off half of the mixture for the kids and only season the mixture that adults will be eating.

Rainbow Wraps

Prep: 10 minutes
Serves 4

4 wholemeal wraps
4 tbsp hummus or 150 g/5 oz
  shredded cooked chicken breast
45 g/1¾ oz Cheddar cheese, grated
1 large carrot, peeled and coarsely
  grated
60 g/2½ oz red cabbage, coarsely
  grated
125 g/4½ oz little gem lettuce,
  shredded
8 cherry tomatoes on the vine,
  quartered
olive oil, for drizzling
sea salt and freshly ground black
  pepper

For first-stage weaning:
Serve the wraps deconstructed,
with the grated veg, a spoonful
of hummus and the wrap sliced
into strips.

For older children:
Older children will enjoy these
as they are, but reserve any
seasoning and olive oil for the
adult portions.

This is a really fun lunch-making activity for the
kids, who will love to get involved packing their own
wraps. It is really colourful and full of the good-for-
you ingredients. You can include any other extra salad
ingredients that you have in the fridge, such as some
sliced peppers or half a boiled egg. I like to keep this
veggie, but you could also add some chicken. They also
make a healthy and convenient lunch box option.

Lay the wraps flat on a board and spread each with
a tablespoon of hummus, if using. Arrange the filling
ingredients on each wrap, making neat strips each of the
cheese, carrot, cabbage, lettuce, tomatoes and chicken, if
using, then drizzle a little olive oil over any adult portions and
season with salt and pepper. Arranging the fillings in this way
will create a pleasing rainbow effect that your kids will love!

Roll up the wraps, then cut each one in half. These are now
ready to serve, but will keep well in the fridge or packed away
in a lunch box until later in the day.

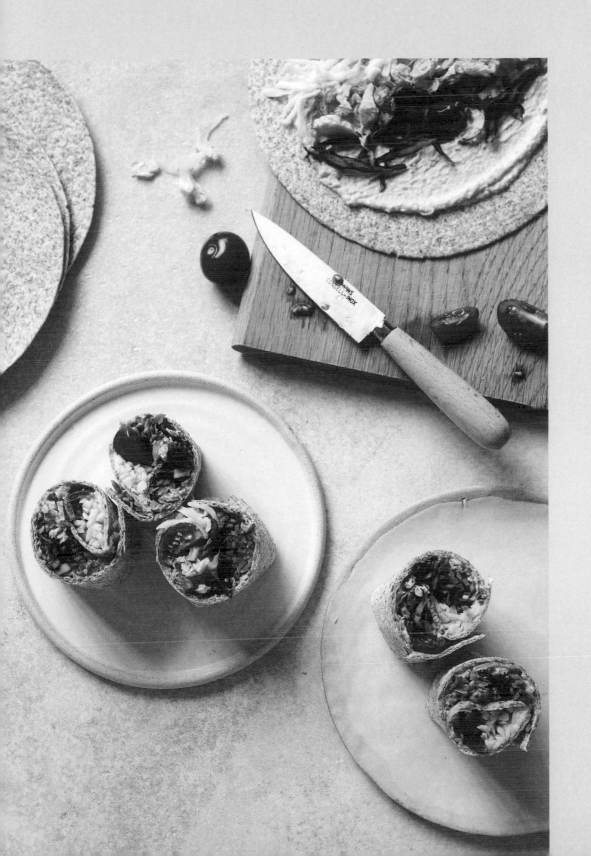

Leftover Roast Chicken & Veggie Soup

Prep: 5 minutes
Cook: 35 minutes
Serves 4

1 tbsp olive oil
2 onions, finely chopped
1 garlic clove, crushed
2 large carrots, peeled and roughly
    chopped
3 sprigs thyme, leaves picked
1.4 litres/2¼ pints chicken stock
200 g/7 oz frozen peas
300 g/10 oz leftover greens, roughly
    chopped (broccoli, cabbage,
    spinach and brussels sprouts all
    work well)
200g/7 oz leftover roast chicken,
    shredded
sea salt and freshly ground black
    pepper
crusty buttered bread, for dunking

For first-stage weaning:
Substitute the stock for water
or low-sodium chicken stock.
Remove and blend some of
the soup before you add the
seasoning. You could also blend
any leftover cooked veggies from
the roast to make a purée.

For older children:
Older children will enjoy this as
it is, just leave any seasoning
until the end and pass it round
to the adults only so that they
can season their own food.

We always cook a roast on a Sunday and if there is
some leftover veg, I will make this soup with it. It is a
one-pot and has all the comforting flavours of
a traditional roast. This is soul food at its best and is
delicious dished up with chunky bread on the side.

Heat the olive oil in a large pan over a medium heat. Add
the onion, garlic, carrots and thyme, and cook, stirring
occasionally, for 15 minutes until the carrots are soft and
onions are golden.

Add the chicken stock to the pan and stir to combine. Bring
the mixture to the boil, then reduce the heat to a simmer
and leave to cook for 15 minutes.

Add the peas, leftover green veg and shredded, cooked
chicken to the pan and stir to combine. Season with salt and
pepper to taste, then leave to cook for 5 minutes.

If you like a chunky soup, ladle half of the soup into a blender
and blend until smooth, then return to the pan with the
unblended soup. If you like your soup smoother, blend all of
the soup in batches to your preferred consistency.

Ladle the soup into bowls and serve with buttered crusty
bread alongside for dunking.

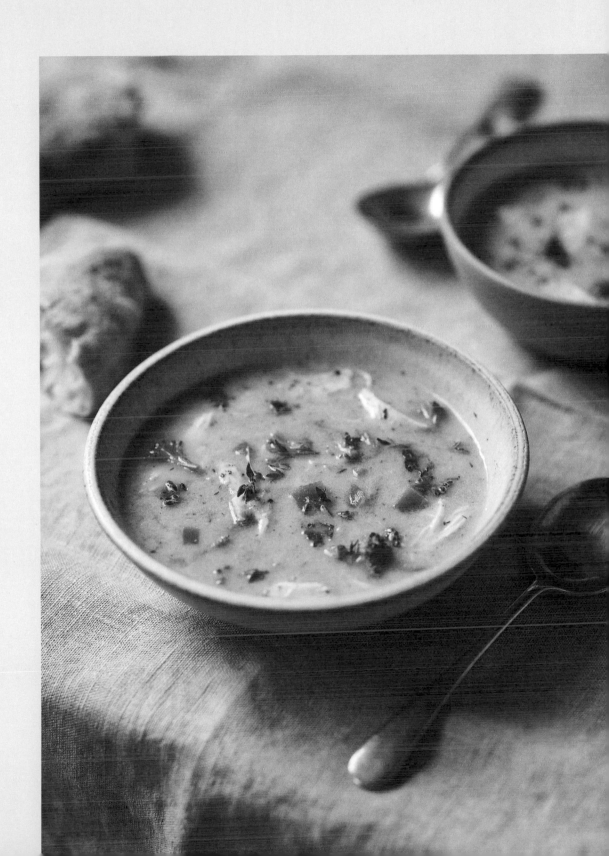

No-Cream, Cream of Tomato Soup

Prep: 10 minutes
Cook: 40 minutes
Serves 8 (or 4 and 4 for the freezer)

2 kg/4½ lbs mixed tomatoes, ideally
  on the vine, halved
3 tbsp olive oil, plus extra for drizzling
10 g/¼ oz fresh thyme (about
  ½ bunch)
1 onion, finely chopped
5 garlic cloves, crushed
1 large bunch basil, leaves picked,
  stalks finely chopped
1 x 400 g/14 oz can plum tomatoes
600 ml/1 pint chicken or vegetable
  stock
4 tbsp green pesto
sea salt and freshly ground black
  pepper
grated fresh Parmesan, to serve

For first-stage weaning:
Blend the roasted tomatoes
with some cooked pasta or rice
to make a purée.

For older children:
The soup can be served as it is
to older children.

Everyone in our house loves soup, especially the extra creamy ones. This soup recipe is so rich and delicious, but does not actually contain any cream, so is good if you are avoiding dairy. It has an amazing bright red colour, so make sure you are not wearing white when you blend it up! This makes enough for four portions to eat and four for the freezer.

Preheat the oven to 200°C/400°F/gas mark 6 and line a roasting tin with foil.

Arrange the tomatoes, cut-side up, in the roasting tin and drizzle over 2 tablespoons of the olive oil. Season with salt and pepper and arrange the whole thyme sprigs over the top of the tomatoes, then transfer to the oven and cook for 30 minutes until the tomatoes are soft.

Meanwhile, heat the remaining tablespoon of oil in a large pan over a medium heat. Add the onions and garlic and cook, stirring continuously, for 5 minutes until soft and translucent. Add the basil leaves and stalks to the pan and stir to combine.

Remove and discard the thyme stalks from the roasted tomatoes, then add the tomatoes to the pan with onions, garlic and basil. Tip in the can of plum tomatoes as well as the stock, breaking up the tomatoes with a wooden spoon as you add them. Bring the mixture to the boil, then reduce to a simmer and leave to cook for 10 minutes.

Remove the pan from the heat and use a stick blender to blend the soup until smooth. Spoon the soup into 4 serving bowls (remembering that half of soup should be left to cool, then frozen for another day), then swirl each bowl with a tablespoon of pesto. Serve the soup hot, with a little grated Parmesan and a drizzle of olive oil, if you like.

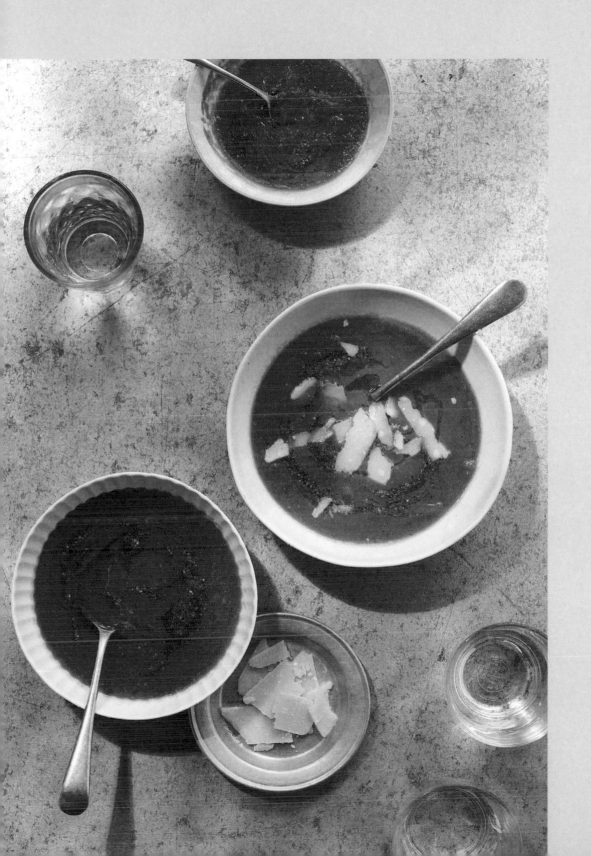

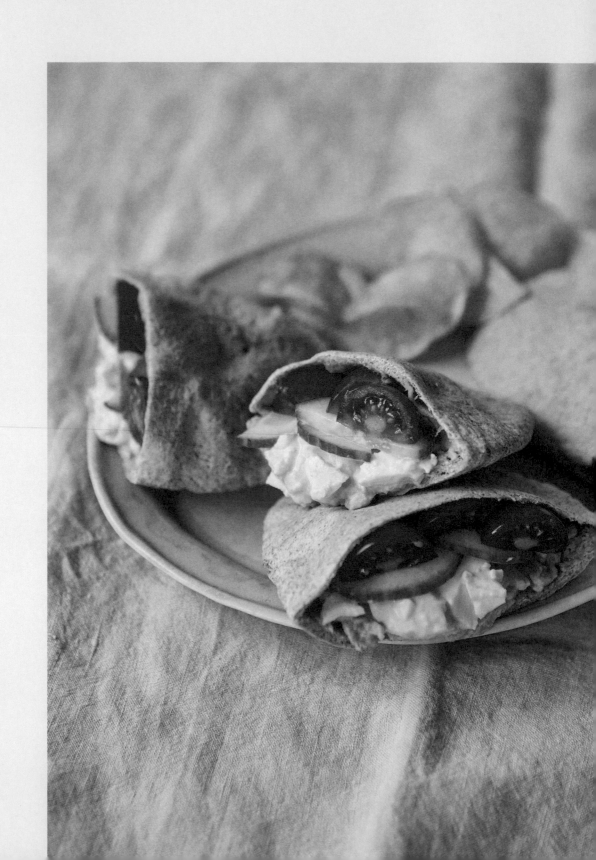

Egg Mayo Pitta Pockets

This egg mayo recipe is super-easy to make and offers a combination of healthy fats, protein and carbohydrates to keep everyone going until dinnertime. The filling for these can be made in advance and stored in the fridge for up to three days.

Bring a pan of water to the boil over a high heat, then reduce to a simmer and carefully add the eggs. Cook for 8 minutes, then drain through a colander and place under a cold running tap for a couple of minutes to cool down.

Peel the eggs, then roughly chop and put in a bowl with the mayonnaise. Mash the eggs and mayonnaise together with a fork, then season with salt and pepper and stir to combine.

Add the chopped avocado to a separate bowl, season with salt and pepper and mash with a fork until almost smooth.

Lightly toast the pitta breads, then slice them open, being careful of any escaping steam.

Spread the avocado over the base of the insides of the pitta breads, then top with the egg mayo mixture. Add the halved cherry tomatoes and sliced cucumber, and serve.

Prep: 5 minutes
Cook: 8 minutes
Serves 4

3 large eggs
3 tbsp mayonnaise
1 ripe avocado, peeled, stoned and roughly chopped
4 wholemeal pitta breads
8 cherry tomatoes, halved
85 g/3 oz cucumber, halved and sliced
sea salt and freshly ground black pepper

For first-stage weaning
Blend some hard-boiled egg with some of the chopped avocado to a purée, then serve with sliced pitta bread and cucumber batons for dunking. You could also cut a hard-boiled egg into wedges and serve it as a finger food alongside.

For older children:
Older children will enjoy these as they are.

Building Positive Foodies: Tips on Talking about Food

I want my kids to have a really positive relationship with food and I've found that the way that I talk about it is important in building that relationship. Children are like sponges and absorb everything that we adults say. Food should never be seen as good, bad, or some form of punishment, so keep your messaging positive and you will have a household of flourishing foodies in no time.

Never label good or bad:

I try to tell my kids that all food is equal, but some types of food should only be eaten occasionally and others can be enjoyed every day. I try to talk about food in terms of what it can offer our bodies, so oranges have vitamin C that can help us fight off germs, fish has omega 3s that are good for our brains and will help us learn, while wholegrains like porridge and beans help your body stay fuller so you have energy for longer.

Be a food explorer:

Teach your child to investigate the foods that they are eating and to think carefully about them and explore them with different senses. Ask them questions like: What colour is it? What does it smell like? What does it feel like? What happens if...? If the food is one that your child is being picky about, this can help them feel more comfortable with the idea of trying it.

Give options:

Sometimes there is no amount of persuasion that will get your child to eat something. Occasionally I will offer a choice of different healthy options at one meal, and let them choose. For example, I might cook carrots, peas, and broccoli and ask which two they might like. Also, let them say 'no, thank you' if they don't want to try something and try again another time. Keep trying, as their tastebuds change over time, so something that they have previously turned down might become a new favourite later on. Alaia used to absolutely hate salmon, but I just kept going with it and now she loves it.

Get them involved:

My kids love to get involved in cooking and I have always tried to let them do something, however small, to make them feel like they are part of it.

Talk about appetite:

Rather than finishing everything on their plates, I always aim for my kids to stop eating when they are full. I tell them that they don't have to eat it all and to always stop when their tummies are full. Similarly, rather than loading up their plates for them, I like to put the food in the middle of the table and let them help themselves. This gives them ownership of their meal and helps them connect to their own appetite with what's plated up in front of them.

Be body positive:

We all have days when we are feeling bloated or not our best, but I always try to use body positive language. I want them to celebrate their own bodies and their friends' bodies. I talk to them about how their bodies are amazing and let them do things like dance and jump high.

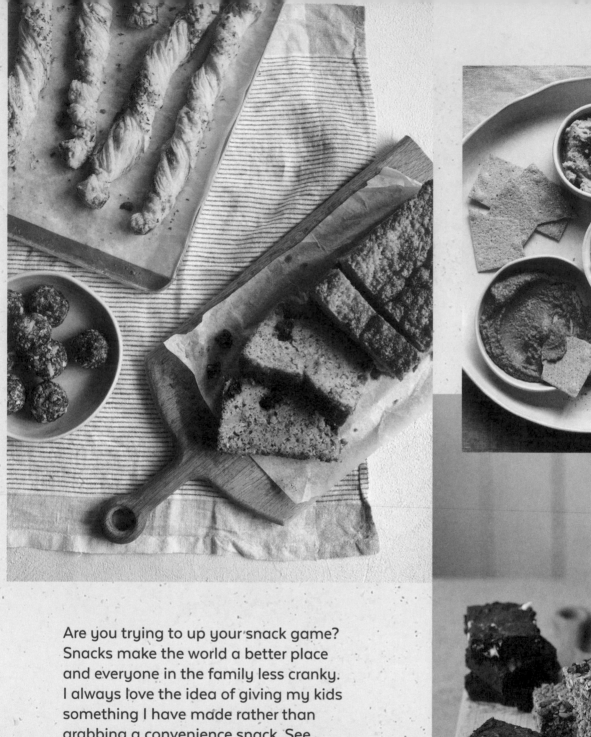

Are you trying to up your snack game? Snacks make the world a better place and everyone in the family less cranky. I always love the idea of giving my kids something I have made rather than grabbing a convenience snack. See classic and fun treats like Best Brownies (see page 104) and Apricot Flapjacks (see page 107), as well as more savoury and healthy ideas like Chia Seed Bites (see page 112) and Cheese & Herb Straws (see page 115).

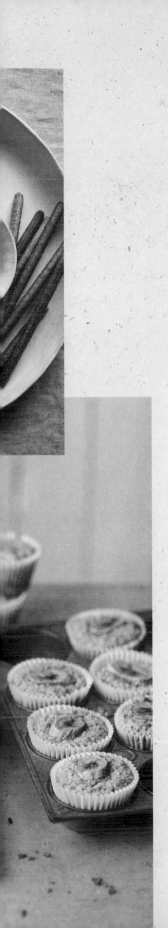

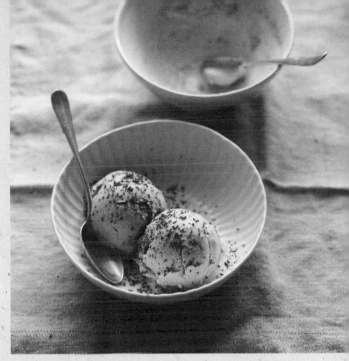

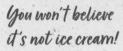
You won't believe it's not ice cream!

Afternoon Snacks

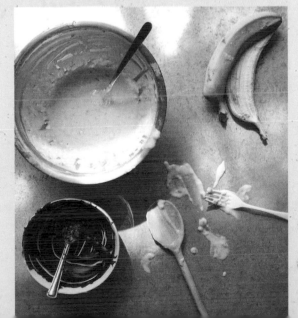

Don't forget to lick the spoon!

Rainy Day & No-Mess Baking

Baking has always been a hit with my children. We baked loads during the lockdowns of 2020 and 2021 and, for me, the less mess the better! If you are looking for simple, easy-to-make recipes that won't leave your kitchen a state, here are some simple, tasty ideas.

Best Brownies

   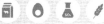

Prep: 5 minutes
Cook: 25 minutes
Makes 16

180 g/6 oz dark chocolate
120 g/4½ oz unsalted butter
200 g/7 oz golden caster sugar
3 large eggs
50 g/1¾ oz sultanas or raisins
120 g/4½ oz plain flour
50 g/1¾ oz white or milk chocolate, cut into chunks

For first-stage weaning:
Sorry kids – this one's not for you!

For older children:
Older children will love these brownies as an occasional treat or as a dessert served with fruit.

I have tried many different classic brownie recipes over the years and this is my favourite. These brownies are so scrumptious and gooey and I love the combination of dark chocolate and raisins. Crispy around the edges and fudgy in the middle, you will not want to share!

Preheat the oven to 180°C/350°F/gas mark 4 and grease a square 20-cm/8-in baking pan with butter and line with greaseproof paper.

Bring a pan half-filled with water to a gentle simmer, then place a heatproof bowl over the top and add the dark chocolate and butter, stirring until completely melted. Remove the bowl from the pan, being careful of escaping steam as you do so, and place on the kitchen counter for a couple of minutes to cool slightly.

Once the chocolate mixture has cooled, stir through the sugar, then crack in and stir through the eggs one at a time. Add the sultanas and stir through, then sift in the flour and stir again until fully incorporated. Fold through the chunks of milk or white chocolate, then pour the mixture into the prepared baking pan and level out the top.

Transfer to the oven and bake for 18–20 minutes until set around the edges but with a slight wobble in the centre. Rest for 20 minutes in the pan, then carefully remove and cut into 16 squares. Serve warm or cooled to room temperature.

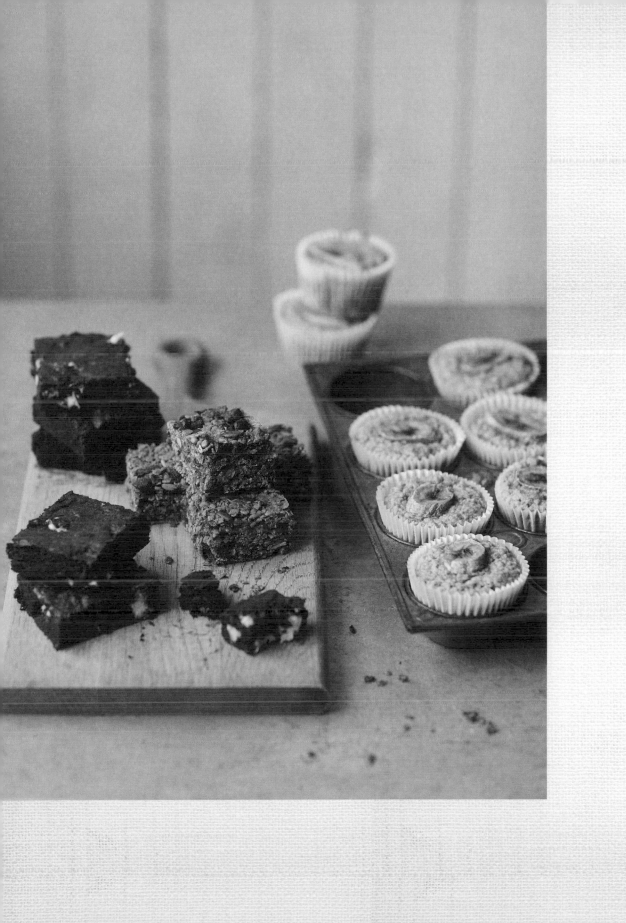

Oaty Banana Mini Muffins

Prep: 10 minutes
Cook: 12 minutes
Makes 40 mini muffins or
   16 larger muffins

250 g/9 oz porridge oats
100 g/3½ oz golden caster sugar
2 tsp baking powder
pinch of salt
50 g/2 oz sultanas or raisins
3 ripe bananas
100 g/3½ oz olive oil or melted
   butter
175 ml/6 fl oz semi-skimmed milk

For first-stage weaning:
Because these contain sugar,
they are unsuitable for children
under 12 months old.

For older children:
These can be enjoyed as they are
and make great snacks, lunch-
box fillers or desserts.

Great for active kids (and adults!), these mini muffins are a fantastic tea-time treat. This is a really good recipe to cook with the kids and can also be made vegan using oil instead of butter and dairy-free milk. These are also a great lunch-box choice – so you can make an extra-large batch of mini muffins and freeze them. If you grab them out of the freezer in the morning then they'll be defrosted by lunch-time.

Preheat the oven to 180°C/350°F/gas mark 4 and line 2 mini-muffin tins or 1 large muffin tin with paper cases.

Put the oats into the bowl of a food processor and blitz to a fine, flour-like consistency, then transfer to a large mixing bowl along with the sugar, baking powder, salt and sultanas or raisins.

If you are making large muffins, cut half of 1 of the bananas into slices and set aside. If you are making mini muffins, chop half of 1 of the bananas into smaller pieces. Put the remaining 2½ bananas into a bowl and mash with a fork until smooth. Add the oil or melted butter and milk and stir to combine, then pour the mixture into the bowl with the dry ingredients and gently fold together until just combined.

Divide the mixture between the prepared cupcake cases, then top each with a little of the sliced or chopped banana. Transfer to the oven and bake for 10–12 minutes for mini muffins, or 18–20 minutes for larger muffins. Either way, the muffins should be golden, well-risen and an inserted skewer should come out clean. Leave the muffins to cool on a wire rack and serve cooled or still slightly warm.

Apricot Flapjacks

Everyone adores flapjacks! These have a really crunchy texture because of the seeds and just the right amount of chew. The seeds also add extra vitamins, minerals and fibre. The apricots and apple add an additional fruity twist. These are also ideal for picnics and walks when every is flagging and needs a pick-me-up on the way home – the first rule of parenthood is to NEVER to leave the house without decent snacks!

Preheat the oven to 170°C/340°F/gas mark 3½ and grease a square 20-cm/8-inch cake pan with butter and line with greaseproof paper.

Put the butter, golden syrup and sugar in pan over a medium heat and cook, stirring occasionally until the butter has melted and the sugar has dissolved.

Meanwhile, pile the grated apple onto the centre of clean tea towel, then bring up the sides to enclose the fruit. Working over a sink or large bowl, twist the base of the tea towel as tightly as you can to remove any excess water from the apple. Add the apple to the pan along with the chopped dried apricots and stir to combine, then remove the pan from heat and stir through the porridge oats and mixed seeds.

Tip the mixture into the prepared baking pan and level out the surface, then transfer to the oven and bake for 40 minutes, or until firm and golden. Set aside to cool in the tin for 25 minutes, then lift out of the baking tin and cut into 12 equal pieces. These will keep in an airtight container for up to 5 days.

Prep: 5 minutes
Cook: 40 minutes
Makes 12

150 g/5½ oz unsalted butter
150 g/5½ oz golden syrup
150 g/5½ oz dark brown sugar
1 apple, peeled, cored and coarsely grated
100 g/3½ oz dried apricots, roughly chopped
300 g/10½ oz porridge oats
1 heaped tbsp mixed seeds (sunflower and pumpkin seeds work well)

For first-stage weaning:
Because these contain sugar, they are unsuitable for children under 12 months old.

For older children:
Older children will love these as they are, served as an occasional treat or with fruit and yoghurt as a dessert.

Hummus – Three Ways

Prep: 10 minutes
Serves 4

3 x 400 g/14 oz cans chickpeas,
  drained
1 garlic clove, crushed
1 tbsp tahini
juice of 2 lemons
150 g/5½ oz extra-virgin olive oil
100 g/3½ oz roasted red peppers
  from a jar
150 g/5½ oz roasted butternut
  squash
sea salt and freshly ground black
  pepper
wholemeal pitta breads and
  chopped veggies of your choice,
  to serve

For first-stage weaning:
Omit the salt from the hummus
and serve with chunky batons
of veg and wedges of pitta bread
for your child to dip.

For older children:
Older children can enjoy the
hummus as it is.

Hummus is such a great snack choice for children and this recipe is packed with nutritional goodness and extra flavour. It is ideal for dipping veggies into, or can be put into a wrap. Tahini is a paste made from sesame seeds and can be found in the supermarket.

Put the drained chickpeas, garlic, tahini and lemon juice in a food processor, then, with the motor running, slowly pour in the olive oil. Process the hummus until smooth, adding a splash of water to loosen if required. Season to taste, then spoon two-thirds of the hummus into a bowl and set aside for later.

Dry the red peppers on some kitchen paper to soak up any excess oil, then add them to the processor with the remaining third of the hummus mixture. Process the hummus again until smooth, then taste and adjust the seasoning if required and spoon the pepper hummus into a bowl.

Rinse and dry the bowl of the food processor, then return half of the plain hummus to the food processor along with the roasted butternut squash. Process the hummus again until smooth, then taste and adjust the seasoning if required and spoon the squash hummus into a bowl.

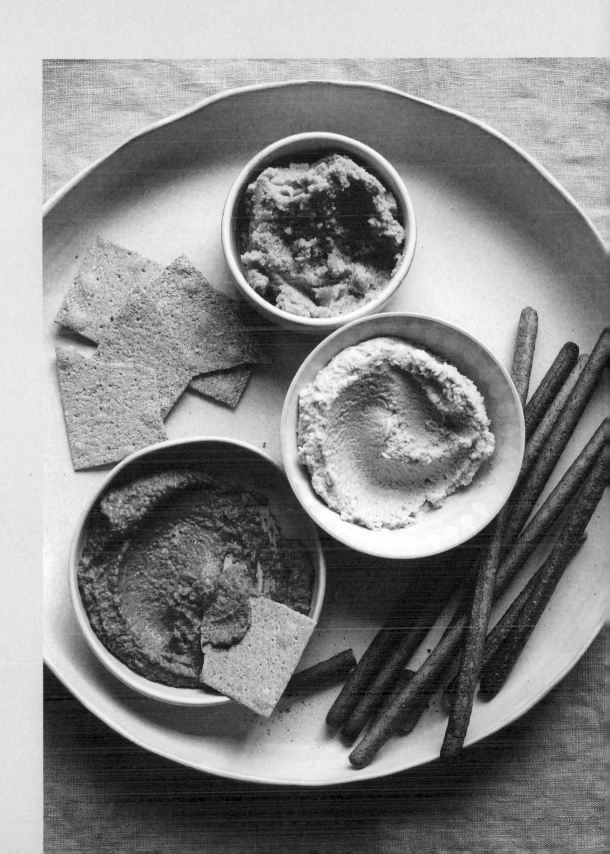

Quick Frozen Banana 'Ice' Cream

Prep: 5 minutes
Serves 4

3 frozen bananas, peeled and sliced
110 g/4 oz Greek yoghurt
5 g/⅛ oz dark chocolate, grated

First-stage weaning:
Weaning babies and young children can enjoy the 'ice' cream without the chocolate.

For older children:
Older children can enjoy the 'ice' cream as it is.

For this recipe, you need frozen bananas – we always have a few ready to go in the freezer but you can also buy frozen ones. This recipe is such a great alternative to 'normal' ice cream because it has the same creamy texture, but is also very healthy. It will even count towards your five a day! By adding some chocolate on top, it feels like a real treat.

Put the banana and yoghurt into the bowl of a food processor or high-powered blender and blend until smooth and creamy. Divide the mixture between serving bowls and sprinkle over a little grated chocolate to serve.

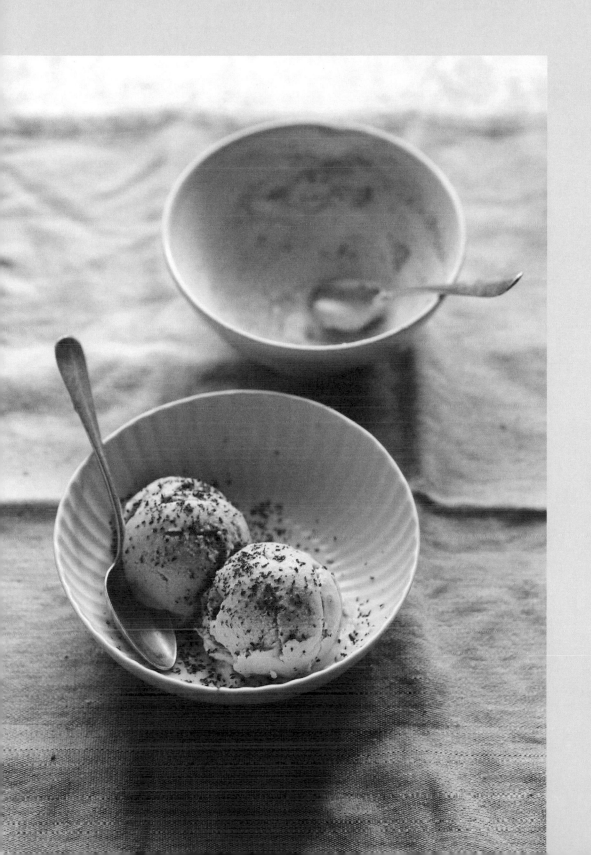

School Pick Up Snack Heroes

My kids are starving after school and when I pick them up, which snack I have brought with me is always one of the first things they will ask me. It's hard to find something that will take the edge off before dinner without completely filling them up, but these recipes do just that!

Chia Seed Bites

Prep: 5 minutes
Makes 20

3 tbsp chia seeds
90 ml/3½ fl oz warm water
125 g/4½ oz porridge oats
100 g/3½ oz almond butter
50 g/1¾ oz sultanas
1 small apple, peeled, cored and grated
4 tbsp clear honey

For first-stage weaning:
Cut in half and serve as a finger food or as part of a meal. Chia seeds are very high in fibre and may have a laxative effect, so introduce in small amounts.

For older children:
Older children can enjoy the bites as they are.

Children will love to help with this simple recipe with mixing and rolling the balls. It is also no-cook, so ideal when you need a quick and nutritious snack. Chia seeds pack a powerful punch – they are rich in fibre, iron, antioxidants, minerals and omega-3 fatty acids. Keep hunger at bay with a couple of these.

Put the chia seeds in a small bowl with the warm water and set aside to thicken for 10 minutes.

Meanwhile put the almond butter, sultanas and half of the porridge oats into the bowl of a food processor and process until the mixture comes together. Spoon the mixture into a bowl along with the remaining oats, the grated apple and the honey. Drain the chia seeds, then add them to the bowl. Give the mixture a good mix until everything is well combined.

Using your hands, roll the mixture into 20 golf ball-sized balls, setting them on a line plate or baking sheet as you make them. Transfer the balls to the fridge for at least 10 minutes before serving. These will keep in the fridge for several days, just grab one straight from the fridge whenever you need an energy boost.

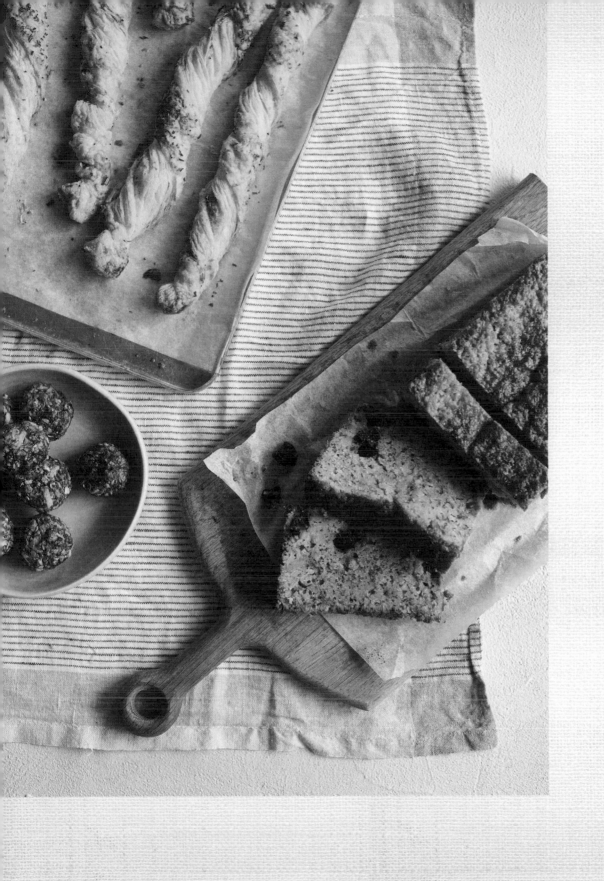

Banana and Blueberry Loaf

Prep: 10 minutes
Cook: 50 minutes
Serves 10

150 g/5½ oz unsalted butter
150 g/5½ oz golden caster sugar
2 large eggs, beaten
splash of milk
3 ripe bananas
150 g/5½ oz self-raising flour
1 heaped tsp baking powder
150 g/5½ oz fresh blueberries

For first-stage weaning:
If making this for babies who are weaning, omit the sugar and blueberries from the mixture. The bananas will still give the loaf a natural sweetness.

For older children:
Older children can enjoy the loaf as it is.

Who didn't make a banana bread over any of the lockdowns? Well, this is a super-simple one, which I made a lot and the kids loved it. It's great for using up over-ripe bananas. You can mix it up using different berries if you would like, or even chunks of chocolate. It always gives great results and is perfect with a cup of tea after the school run!

Preheat the oven to 160°C/325°F/gas mark 3 and grease a 900 g/2 lb loaf tin with butter and line with greaseproof paper.

Using a stand mixer or an electric whisk, beat the butter and sugar until pale and fluffy. Crack the eggs in one at a time, beating to incorporate between each addition. Add a splash of milk and beat again to combine.

Peel and mash 2 of the bananas with a fork until smooth, then add to the bowl with a couple of tablespoons of the flour and beat again until combined. Sift in the remaining flour and baking powder, then beat until combined. Add most of the blueberries and gently fold through the mixture, being careful not to break the fruit.

Pour the mixture into the prepared cake tin and level out with a wooden spoon or spatula. Peel the remaining banana and cut in half lengthways, then lay the banana halves, cut-side up, along the top of the batter and sprinkle over the remaining blueberries. Transfer to the oven for 45–50 minutes until golden, well-risen and an inserted skewer comes out clean.

Leave to cool in the tin for 15 minutes, then turn the loaf out onto a wire rack and cool to room temperature before slicing and serving. This will keep for several days in an airtight container.

Cheese & Herb Straws

Flaky, flavoursome and crisp, cheese straws always go down a storm with the kids after school, at kids' parties and I will often serve them when we have friends here for drinks or dinner. They're yummy on their own but also great for dipping!

Prep: 5 minutes
Cook: 10 minutes
Makes 14

375 g/13 oz ready-rolled puff pastry
40 g/1½ Parmesan cheese, grated
2 sprigs rosemary, leaves finely
   chopped
olive oil, for drizzling

Preheat the oven to 200°C/400°F/gas mark 6 and line a baking sheet with greaseproof paper.

Unroll the puff pastry on its lining paper on the kitchen counter and scatter over most of the Parmesan and all of the chopped rosemary leaves, then drizzle a little olive oil over the top.

Set the pastry in front of you in landscape orientation, and using a sharp knife or pizza cutter, cut the pastry top to bottom into 14 equal strips, each roughly 2 cm/¾ inches wide. Hold the pastry strips at opposite ends and twist in alternate directions to create decorative twists. Lay the twists on the prepared baking tray and sprinkle over the remaining grated Parmesan.

Transfer the tray to the oven and bake the twists for 10–12 minutes until crisp and golden. Transfer to a wire rack and leave to cool. These will keep for a few days in an airtight container.

For first-stage weaning:
These can be offered to weaning children as they are.

For older children:
Older children can enjoy the bites as they are.

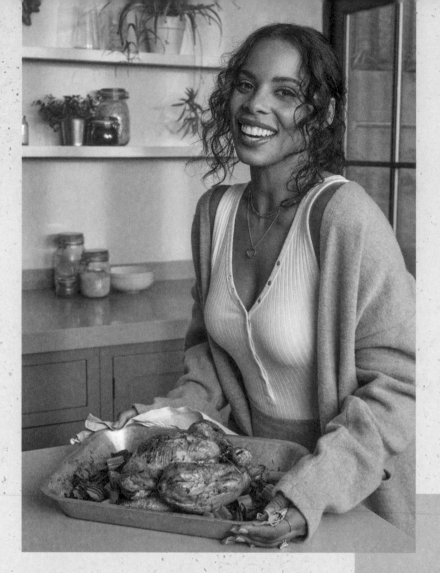

My kids are always starving when they come home from school, so I like to have the dinner on the table as quickly as possible. Whether you are looking for something fast and nutritious that you can cook with your eyes shut (try my One-Pot Veggie, Bean & Quinoa Stew on page 152) or something that can you prepare in advance and freeze like Cottage Pie (see page 123), dinner does not have to be a chore. If you are vegetarian or trying to cut down on meat, I have tried to add veggie alternatives to many of these recipes so that they can easily be adapted to suit your diet.

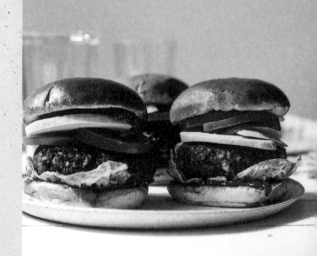

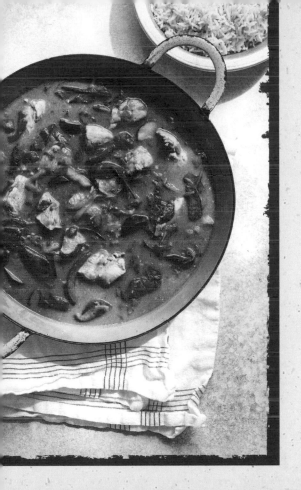

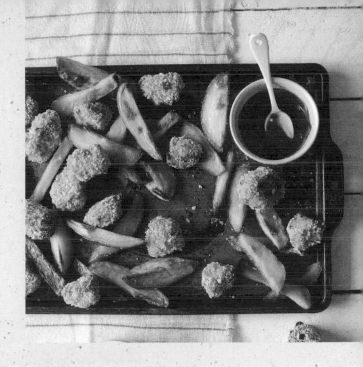

Dinner

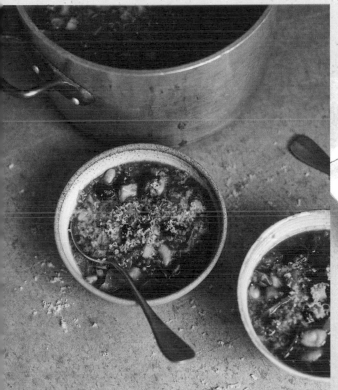

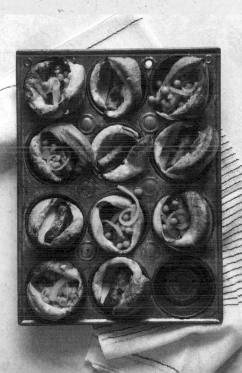

Cute and delicious!

Spicy Chicken (or Tofu) Curry in a Hurry

Prep: 5 minutes
Cook: 25 minutes
Serves 8 (or 4 and 4 for the freezer)

1 tbsp olive oil
1 red onion, halved and finely sliced
2 garlic cloves, crushed
1 courgette, cut into 2 cm/¾ in pieces
1 red pepper, deseeded and sliced
400 g/14 oz chicken breast or tofu
2 tbsp korma curry paste (check label
   for allergens)
1 small bunch coriander, leaves
   picked and stalks finely chopped
1 x 400 g/14 oz can chopped
   tomatoes
1 x 400 ml/14 fl oz can coconut milk
handful of spinach leaves
sea salt and freshly ground black
   pepper
cooked basmati rice and mango
   chutney, to serve

For first-stage weaning:
Pre-made curry pastes can
be quite salty, so are best
avoided for very young children.
Instead, cook of some of the veg
in a separate pan until tender,
then blitz up with some yoghurt
and cooked basmati rice to make
a purée.

For older children:
Serve the curry as it is, but with
a little yoghurt stirred through to
cool it down for younger palates.

I've always tried to introduce spice to my kids from an early age, and this crowd-pleasing curry is a dish that all of the family can eat together. I've also included a tofu option for those who don't eat meat, which has a similar meaty texture to chicken. This makes a big batch, so is perfect for portioning off half to put in the freezer for another day.

Heat the oil in a large pan over a medium heat. Add the red onion, garlic, courgette and red pepper and cook, stirring occasionally, for 5 minutes until softened.

Meanwhile, chop the chicken or tofu into bite-sized chunks, then add to the pan along with the curry paste and chopped coriander stalks. Cook, stirring continuously, for 5 minutes to seal the chicken, then add the chopped tomatoes and coconut milk and stir to combine. Bring the mixture to the boil, then reduce to a simmer and leave to cook for 10 minutes, stirring occasionally until the sauce is fragrant and the chicken is cooked through.

Stir through the spinach until wilted, then season the curry with salt and pepper to taste, spoon into serving bowls and serve hot, with cooked basmati rice and mango chutney alongside and a scattering of coriander leaves over the top.

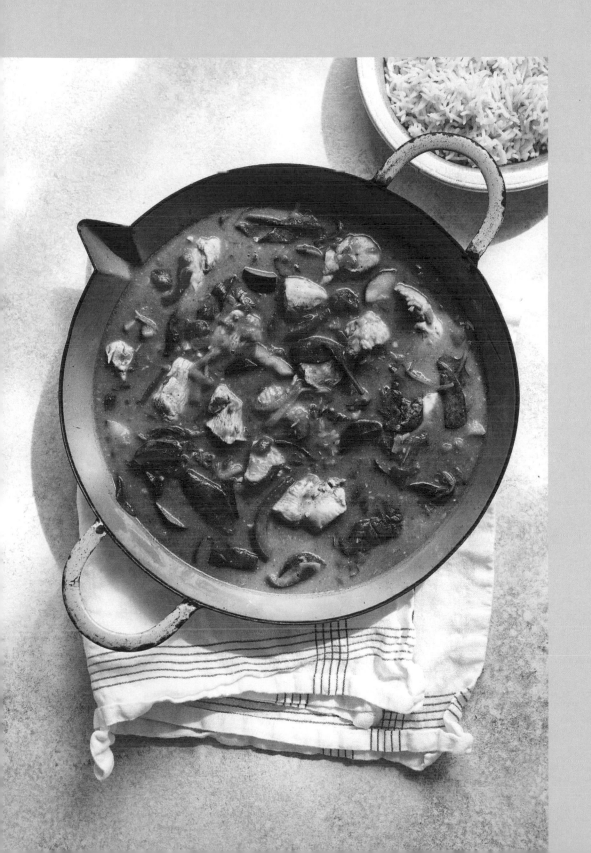

Sausage & Bean Casserole

Prep: 25 minutes
Cook: 10 minutes
Serves 4

2 tbsp olive oil
1 small bunch thyme, leaves picked
1 stick celery, cut into 2 cm/¾ in pieces
1 carrot, peeled and finely chopped
1 onion, finely chopped
1 courgette cut into 2 cm/¾ in pieces
1 tsp fennel seeds, crushed
6-8 pork or vegetarian sausages
2 x 400 g/14 oz cans plum tomatoes
2 x 400 g cans cannellini or other beans, drained
600 g/1 lb 5 oz potatoes, peeled and cut into 2 cm/¾ in pieces
sea salt and freshly ground black pepper

For first-stage weaning:

Omit the seasoning from the stew and potato, then remove the sausages and blitz some of the vegetables and sauce to a purée. Serve with a little of the mashed potato alongside.

For older children:

Older children will enjoy this as it is, though you could remove the sausages and blitz the sauce until smooth for fussy eaters. Omit the seasoning from the casserole and potatoes and pass around separately to the adults when serving.

How can you go wrong with sausages and beans? This is a great, no-fuss, one-pot meal that is perfect for the colder months. Use any type of beans you have in the cupboard – I love cannellini beans, but any type will do. If I cook sausage and mash and have any sausages left over, I'll cook this casserole the next day.

Heat the oil in a large pan over a medium heat. Add the thyme leaves, celery, carrot, onion, courgette and crushed fennel seeds and cook, stirring, for 5 minutes until the vegetables are starting to soften and caramelize. Add the sausages to the pan and cook, stirring occasionally, for another 5 minutes until they start to take on some colour, then add the canned tomatoes and beans and stir to combine. Refill one of the cans with boiling water, then carefully tip into the pan. Bring the mixture to the boil, then reduce to a simmer and leave to cook, stirring occasionally, for 15–20 minutes until the sausages and vegetables have cooked through and the sauce has thickened.

Meanwhile put the potatoes in a pan and cover with cold water. Place over a medium heat and bring to the boil, then reduce the heat to a simmer and cook for 15–20 minutes until tender. Drain the potatoes through a colander, leave to steam dry for a couple of minutes, then return to the pan, season with salt and pepper, and mash until smooth.

Once the casserole is cooked, season to taste, then ladle into serving bowls and serve hot, with the mashed potatoes alongside.

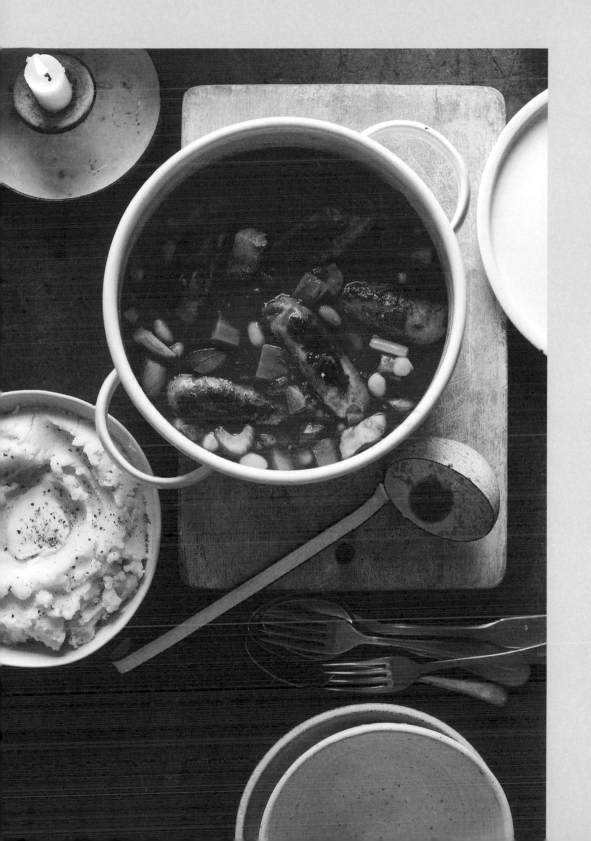

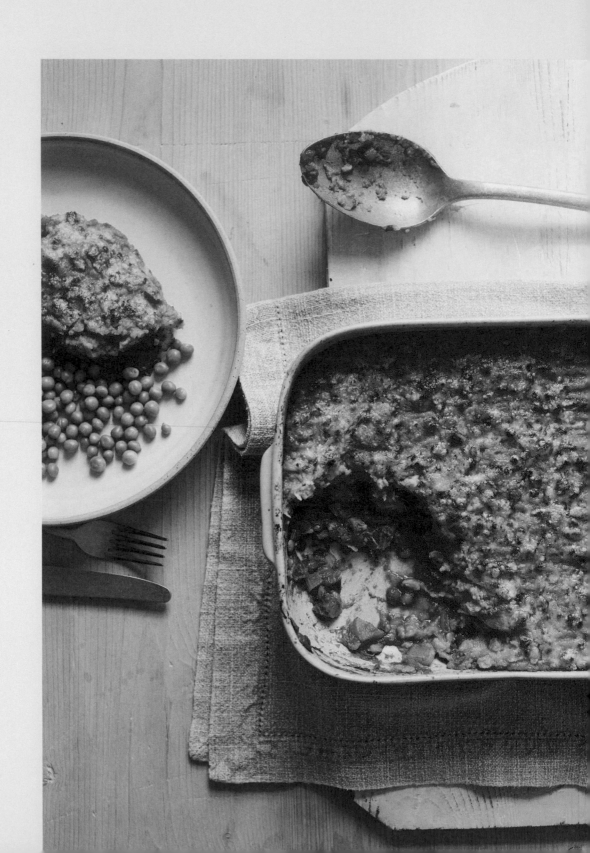

Cottage Pie

This is one of my favourite comfort foods, and such a classic. Rich beef is topped with creamy mash, which is then cooked to perfection. I have included a lentil option for veggies, which is just as hearty and filling. This a long-standing favourite with everyone and also freezes really well, so is perfect for those evenings when I'm too busy or tired to cook.

Put the onion, carrot and celery into a food processor and pulse until finely chopped. Heat the oil in a large pan over a medium heat, then add the finely chopped vegetables, garlic, thyme leaves and minced beef, if using. Cook, stirring occasionally to break the mince down, for 15 minutes until the vegetables are tender and the meat has browned.

Add the tomato purée to the pan and stir to combine, then tip in the chopped tomatoes. Fill the tomato can with boiling water, then carefully pour add to the pan and repeat, so that you have added 2 canfuls of water. If you are using lentils rather than beef, also add these now. Give the mixture a stir to combine, bring to the boil, then reduce to a simmer and leave to cook, covered but stirring occasionally, for 10 minutes, then remove the lid and cook for 10 minutes more. Season to taste.

While the sauce is bubbling, put the potatoes or sweet potatoes in a pan of cold, salted water and place over a high heat. Bring to the boil, then reduce the heat to a simmer and leave to cook for 15 minutes until the potatoes are tender. Drain through a colander and leave to steam dry for a couple of minutes, then return the potatoes to the pan and mash until smooth.

Preheat the grill to high.

Spoon the filling mixture into the base of a large, flameproof baking dish, then spoon over the potatoes, spreading them out in an even layer to cover the filling. Scatter over the grated Cheddar or Parmesan, then place the pie under the grill for 8–10 minutes until golden and bubbling.

Serve the pie hot, spooned into serving bowls and with your choice of steamed green veg alongside.

Prep: 5 minutes
Cook: 40-45 minutes
Serves 4

1 tbsp olive oil
1 onion, quartered
1 large carrot, peeled and roughly chopped
2 celery sticks, roughly chopped
1 garlic clove, crushed
4 sprigs thyme, leaves picked
500 g/1 lb 2 oz lean minced beef or 150 g/5 oz dried red lentils
2 tbsp tomato purée
1 x 400g/14 oz can chopped tomatoes
700 g/1 lb 9 oz sweet or white potatoes, peeled and cut into 2 cm/¾ in pieces
30 g/1 oz Cheddar or Parmesan cheese, grated
sea salt and freshly ground black pepper
cooked peas or steamed broccoli, to serve

For first-stage weaning:
Omit the seasoning when making the pie, then blend a small portion to a purée before serving.

For older children:
Older children can enjoy the pie as it is.

Quick & Easy Stir Fry

Prep: 5 minutes
Cook: 5 minutes
Serves 4

225 g/8 oz firm tofu or frozen king
   prawns
1 tbsp sesame oil
1 red onion, halved and finely sliced
150 g/5 oz chestnut mushrooms,
   sliced
1 red pepper, deseeded, halved and
   finely slice
150 g/5 oz sugar snaps, tenderstem
   broccoli, baby corn or mange tout
   (or a mixture)
250 g/9 oz medium egg noodles
100 g/3½ oz black bean sauce
2 tbsp water

For first-stage weaning:
Simply fry off the vegetables and
prawns or tofu in a little oil, then
purée with some of the cooked
noodles. If using prawns, ensure
they are thoroughly cooked.

For older children:
Older children can enjoy this as
it is. If you're worried about the
salt content in the sauce, you
could heat it separately and pour
over the adult's portions before
serving.

This super-easy stir-fry takes minutes to throw
together and is bursting with flavour. When time
is short during the week, this is one of my go-to
meals. It can be made with prawns or firm tofu. I love
mushrooms, and so do the girls, but leave them out
if your kids aren't keen. There is still plenty of vibrant
crunchy veg in the form of the sugar snaps, tenderstem
and mange tout.

If you are using tofu, cut it into 1 cm/½ inch cubes. Heat the
oil in a large frying pan or wok over a medium heat, then add
the tofu and cook for 2–3 minutes, stirring continuously until
browned on all sides. Keep the pan on the heat, but remove
the tofu with a slotted spoon and set aside. If you are not
using tofu, simply heat the oil as described above and then
continue from here.

Add the sliced onion, mushrooms, pepper and other
vegetables to the pan and cook, stirring continuously for
5 minutes until softened. Add the prawns to the pan, if using,
and cook, stirring, for another 5 minutes.

Meanwhile, cook the noodles in boiling water according to
packet instructions, then drain and tip into the pan along
with the black bean sauce, water and the tofu, if using. Toss
everything to combine, then divide the mixture between
serving plates and serve hot.

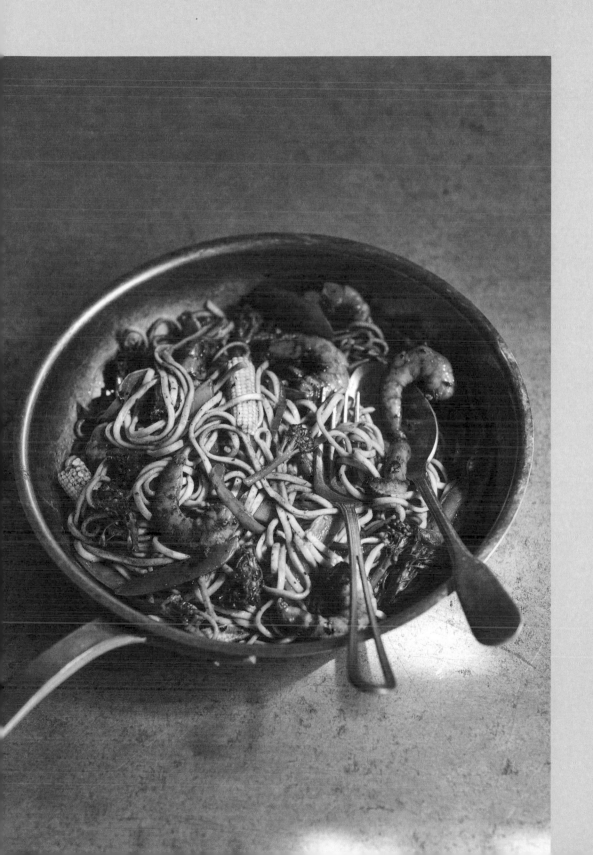

Veggie (or Beef) Bolognese

Prep: 5 minutes
Cook: 40-45 minutes
Serves 4

1 onion, roughly chopped
1 large carrot, peeled and roughly
  chopped
1 celery stick, roughly chopped
1 tbsp olive oil
2 garlic cloves, crushed
large bunch basil, leaves and stalks
  roughly chopped
350 g/12 oz frozen Quorn pieces or
  500 g/1 lb 2 oz lean minced beef
200 ml/7 fl oz red wine
½ tsp ground cinnamon
2 tbsp Worcestershire sauce
2 x 400 g/14 oz cans chopped
  tomatoes
350 g/12 oz wholewheat spaghetti
30 g/1 oz Parmesan cheese, grated

For first-stage weaning:
Omit the wine and seasoning
when making the Bolognese,
then blend some of the sauce
with a little spaghetti to make
a purée.

For older children:
Older children can eat this as it is,
though you may want to cut up
the pasta a little before serving
to make it a bit easier (and less
messy!) to eat.

This is my best Bolognese, which is bursting with
deep flavours from the addition of cinnamon and
Worcestershire sauce. A total classic – it is so easy to
knock up in a hurry and is another great freezer staple.
If you are a veggie, simply swap out the beef for Quorn
pieces and you can enjoy the same delicious flavours.

Put the onion, carrot and celery into a food processor and
pulse until finely chopped. Pick a few leaves from the basil to
use as a garnish and set aside, then roughly chop the rest of
the bunch, stalks and all.

Heat the oil in a large pan over a medium heat, then add
the finely chopped vegetables, garlic and chopped basil.
Cook, stirring continuously for 10 minutes until softened and
starting to caramelize. Add the Quorn pieces or minced beef
and cook stirring and breaking down with a wooden spoon,
for 5 minutes until the Quorn or meat is nicely browned.
Stir the red wine through the mixture and leave to simmer
for 5 minutes.

Add the cinnamon, Worcester sauce and chopped tomatoes
to the pan. Fill one the tomato tins with boiling water, then
carefully pour add to the pan and stir to combine. Bring the
mixture to the boil, then reduce to a simmer and leave to cook
for 20–30 minutes until the Bolognese has thickened. Season
to taste.

While the Bolognese is cooking, bring a large pan of salted
water to the boil over a medium heat. Cook the spaghetti
according to packet instructions, then drain through a
colander reserving some of the pasta water.

Transfer the drained pasta along with a ladleful of pasta
water to the pan with the Bolognese, then give everything
a good stir to ensure that the pasta is well coated with the
sauce. Divide the mixture between serving bowls, scatter with
grated Parmesan and garnish with the reserved basil leaves.
Serve hot.

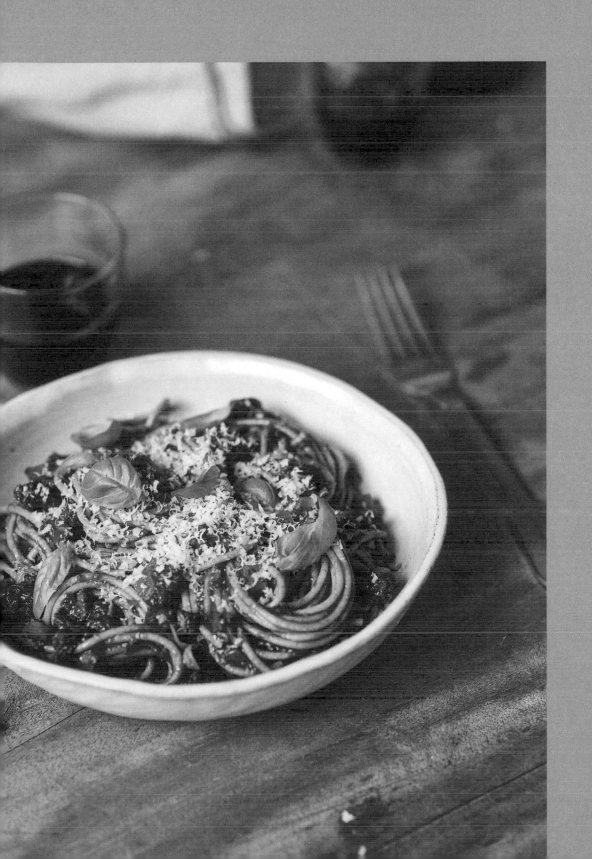

Are you looking for a lasagne recipe to feed a crowd? Meat eaters and veggies alike will be fighting over second helpings of this recipe. I combine red lentils, tomatoes, celery, carrots, and onions to make the filling, and the mozzarella provides a deliciously creamy topping. This can easily be prepared in advance for busy days.

For first-stage weaning:
The filling makes a perfect textured purée for first-stage weaners, simply blitz it up and serve it with cooked baby-shell pasta.

For older children:
For toddlers and pre-schoolers, serve the lentil mix with a little of the cheese sauce drizzled over the top, cooked pasta shapes and some extra grated cheese alongside. For older children, serve the lasagne as is, but cut it into bite-sized morsels for little mouths.

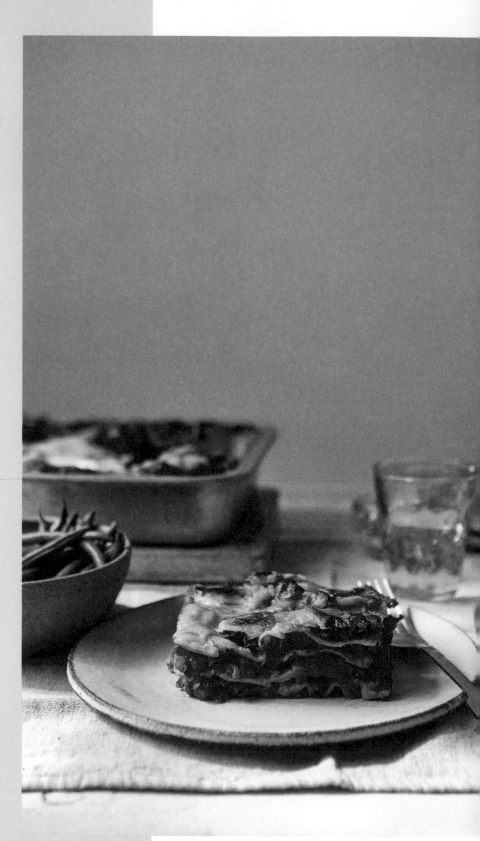

Veggie Lasagne

Heat 1 tablespoon of the olive oil in a large pan over a medium heat. Once hot, add the onion, carrot and celery and cook, stirring occasionally, for 10–15 minutes until soft and translucent.

Add the tomato purée to the pan and stir to combine with the vegetables, then tip in the chopped tomatoes. Fill one of the empty cans with cold water and add that to the pan, then add the lentils and give everything a stir to combine. Bring the mixture to the boil, then reduce the heat to a gentle simmer and leave to cook for 30 minutes, stirring occasionally. While the sauce is cooking, preheat the oven to 200°C/400°F/gas mark 6.

Meanwhile, make the white sauce by heating the butter and a little olive oil in a pan over a medium heat. Once the butter has melted, add the flour to the pan and stir over the heat until the mixture has come together and thickened. Add a little of the milk to the pan and cook, whisking continuously until the liquid thickens. Keep adding more of the milk to the pan, whisking and thickening between each addition until all of the milk has been used up. Add the cheese to the pan and whisk again until the cheese has melted and you have a smooth, glossy sauce.

To assemble the lasagne, set a 20 x 30 cm/8 x 12 inch rectangular baking dish on the counter and ladle a quarter of the tomato and lentil mixture into the dish, spreading it out with the back of the ladle to form an even layer. Add a layer of white sauce over the tomato mixture and dot a quarter of the mozzarella over, then top with a layer of the dried lasagne sheets. Repeat the layers until all of the tomato mixture has been used up and finish with a final layer of white sauce dotted with mozzarella.

Transfer the lasagne to the oven to bake for 30 minutes until golden, bubbling and the lasagne sheets are tender. Serve hot with your choice of steamed green vegetables alongside.

Prep: 40 minutes
Cook: 30 minutes
Serves 4

4 tbsp olive oil
1 large onion, finely chopped
1 large carrot, finely chopped
1 celery stick, finely chopped
2 tbsp tomato purée
2 x 400 g/14 oz cans chopped
  tomatoes
150 g/5 oz dried red lentils
1 x 125 g/4½ oz ball of mozzarella
150 g/5 oz dried lasagne sheets
steamed green vegetables, to serve

For the white sauce:
40 g/1½ oz unsalted butter
olive oil
2 heaped tbsp plain flour
700 ml/1¼ pints semi-skimmed
  milk
75 g/3 oz Cheddar cheese, grated
sea salt and freshly ground black
  pepper

Skills Chart for Rewarding Little Chefs

My girls started wanting to help in the kitchen when they were tiny and have been helping me ever since. They particularly love baking (no surprise there!) with me and helping with basic tasks, such as weighing out ingredients. Valle sits on the worktop next to me and thinks she is so grown up.

I have created this little chart, organized by age, to give you some ideas about how your children can get involved in the kitchen. For each age group, I have started with the simpler tasks and then got steadily more complicated, so that the oldest children in each age bracket will be able to complete the tasks at the bottom of each list. Draw up your own list together with your kids then, as they complete the tasks, give them a tick or, even better, a sticker! Each time you do something new in the kitchen start a new list so there's always an opportunity for more ticks and stickers.

Under 3s:

- Pouring ingredients into a mixing bowl
- Stirring dry ingredients
- Washing fruit and vegetables
- Sprinkling flour
- Mashing soft fruit or potatoes with a masher or fork
- Decorating cakes

Age 3-5:

- Mixing ingredients with a spoon or hands
- Tearing herbs or salad leaves
- Greasing cake tins
- Spreading butter on bread or icing on a cake
- Opening packets

- o Rolling, shaping, and cutting dough
- o Kneading bread dough
- o Breading fish or other ingredients (see my Chicken or Mushroom Nuggets on page 135)

Age 5-7:

- o General helping around the kitchen, such as loading and unloading the dishwasher or tidying items away
- o Weighing ingredients on the scales or in measuring cup
- o Cutting baking parchment with blunt scissors
- o Supervised careful grating
- o Using the microwave for simple tasks
- o Cutting up soft foods, such as butter, with a blunt knife
- o Getting items from the fridge or cupboards
- o Setting the table
- o Getting their own breakfast cereal
- o Using a pizza cutter
- o Peeling hard-boiled eggs
- o Peeling fruit
- o Reading simple recipes and weighing ingredients

Age 8-10:

- o Whisking
- o Making toast
- o Loading and unloading the dishwasher
- o Planning meals
- o Inventing a recipe for a smoothie or fruit salad
- o Slicing vegetables with a butter knife, with supervision
- o Making salads
- o Making pasta, with supervision
- o Using the oven, with supervision
- o Making scrambled eggs, with supervision
- o Following simple, child-friendly recipes

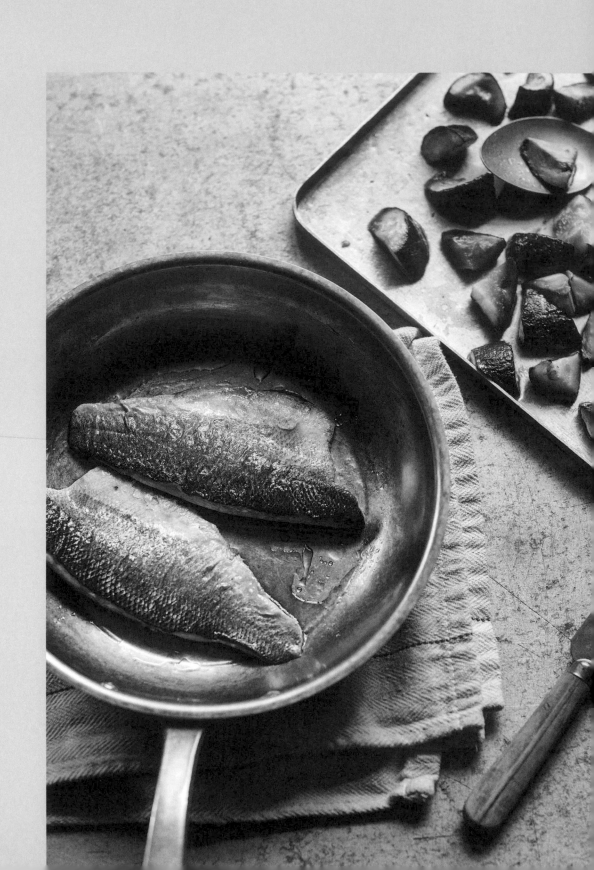

Sea Bass & Courgettes with Coconut Rice

We enjoy eating sea bass because it is so light and naturally quite sweet. I have a fantastic local fishmonger who I like to buy my fish from, but there are great fish sections in most large supermarkets.

Preheat the oven to 180°C/350°F/gas mark 4.

Put the courgettes in a roasting tin and drizzle over the soy sauce, lemon juice and 3 tablespoons of the sesame oil. Transfer to the oven and cook for 30 minutes, giving the tin a shake halfway through cooking until tender and golden.

Meanwhile, prepare the coconut rice. Put the rice in a sieve and rinse under cold running water until the water runs clear. Put the rice in a pan over a medium heat with the boiling water and the can of coconut milk. Bring to the boil, then reduce to a simmer and cover the pan with a lid. Cook for 20 minutes, then turn off the heat and leave to stand, still covered with the lid, for an additional 5 minutes.

Heat the remaining tablespoon of sesame oil in a frying pan over a medium heat. Add the sea bass fillets, skin-side down and cook for 3 minutes until the skin is crisp. Turn over the fillets and cook on the top side for another 2 minutes until the fish is cooked through.

Take the lid off the rice and stir through most of the chopped coriander, then divide the rice between serving plates. Spoon the courgettes over the rice, then top each plate with a sea bass fillet and a sprinkling of coriander. Serve hot.

Prep: 5 minutes
Cook: 30 minutes
Serves 4

4 courgettes (approx. 350 g/12 oz), cut into 2 cm/¾ in pieces
4 tbsp sesame oil
4 tbsp soy sauce
juice of 1 lemon
4 x 100 g/3½ oz sea bass fillets

For the coconut rice:
400 g/14 oz basmati rice
200 ml/7 fl oz boiling water
1 x 400 ml/14 fl oz can coconut milk
1 small bunch coriander, stalks and leaves finely chopped

For first-stage weaning:
Pan-fry some of the courgettes in a little oil, but without any soy until tender. Blitz the cooked courgette with some of the fish and a few tablespoons of the rice to make a purée.

For older children
Older children can enjoy this is as it is. Soy sauce is very salty, so you may want to use a reduced-salt variety.

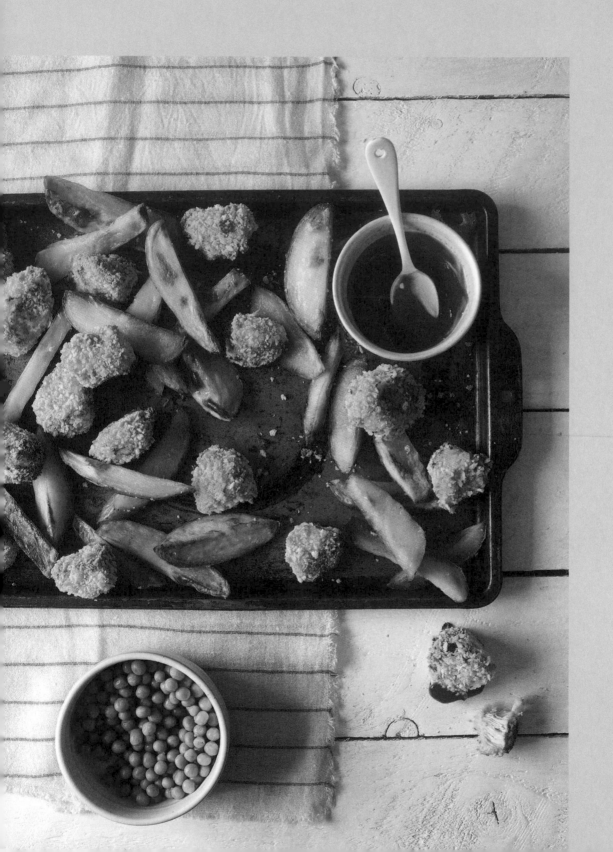

Chicken (or Mushroom) Nuggets with Chips

This homemade chicken nugget recipe is a great alternative to shop-bought versions and is packed with flavour. It is a favourite Friday-night treat meal for my family, and Alaia and Valle like to help dipping the chicken or mushrooms in the flour, eggs and breadcrumbs. Just make sure the kids wash their hands well after handling the chicken. The garlic granules gives these nuggets an extra punchy flavour.

Preheat the oven to 180°C/350°F/gas mark 4 and line 2 baking sheets with foil.

Put the potatoes in a pan and cover with cold water, then place over a medium heat and bring to the boil. Reduce the heat to a gentle simmer, then cook for 4 minutes. Drain the chips through a colander and leave to steam dry for a couple of minutes, then tip onto one of the baking sheets, season with salt and pepper and drizzle with the olive oil. Give everything a mix with your hands to ensure that the chips are well coated with the seasoning and oil, then transfer the tray to the oven for 45–50 minutes until the chips are crisp and golden.

Meanwhile, if you are making your own breadcrumbs, tear the bread into the bowl of a food processor and process until fine. Set three shallow bowls next to each other on your work surface. Working left to right, put the flour in the first bowl, beat the eggs into the second bowl and put the breadcrumbs and garlic granules in the third, mixing so that the breadcrumbs are coated in the garlic granules.

To coat the nuggets, dip a piece of chicken or a mushroom first in the flour to coat, then in the egg and finally in the breadcrumbs. Lay the coated nuggets on the remaining prepared baking sheet and repeat the process with the rest of the chicken or mushrooms.

Transfer the nuggets to the oven for 20–25 minutes until golden brown and cooked through.

Once everything is cooked, divide the nuggets and chips between serving plates and serve with your choice of veg and sauces for dipping alongside.

Prep: 15 minutes
Cook: 50 minutes
Serves 4

800 g/1 lb 12 oz floury potatoes, peeled and cut into 2 cm/¾ in thick chips
2 tbsp olive oil
250 g/9 oz stale wholemeal bread or shop-bought breadcrumbs
100 g/3½ oz plain flour
3 large eggs
2 tsp garlic granules
4 chicken breasts, cut into 4 cm/ 1½ in 'nuggets' or 250 g/9 oz button mushrooms
sea salt and freshly ground black pepper
cooked peas, sweetcorn or baked bean, to serve

For first-stage weaning:
These are unsuitable for first-stage weaning, but older children who are ready for finger foods will love nibbling these.

For older children:
Kids will love this as it is. Omit the seasoning from the chips and pass salt and pepper around to the adults only when serving.

Mini Toad in the Hole

Prep: 10 minutes
Cook: 20 minutes
Serves 4-6

6 tbsp sunflower oil
4 large eggs
140 g/5 oz plain flour, plus 2 tbsp
  for the gravy
200 ml/7 fl oz whole or semi-
  skimmed milk
12 chipolata sausages
2 sprigs fresh rosemary, leaves finely
  chopped
1 onion, halved and finely sliced
100 g/3½ oz frozen peas
1 tsp vegetable bouillon powder
  (check label for allergens)
steamed tenderstem broccoli, to
  serve
sea salt and freshly ground black
  pepper

For first-stage weaning:
When babies are ready for finger
foods, serve them plain Yorkshire
puddings, without the chipolatas
or gravy.

For older children:
Older children will love these
dinky toad in the holes as they
are. Simply omit the seasoning
from the batter mix and try
and use a reduced-salt bouillon
powder when making the gravy.

This easy and delicious meal reminds me of my
childhood, when my mum would always make
steaming tins of toad in the hole. This version has
peas and tenderstem broccoli added for extra veggie
goodness. If you are vegetarian or trying to eat less
meat, simply use vegetarian chipolatas. I like these
mini ones because it is much easier to see how much
the children have eaten and not overwhelm them.

Preheat the oven to 230°C/450°F/gas mark 8 and divide
4 tablespoons of the oil between the holes of 2 x 12-hole
muffin tins. Put the tins in the oven to heat, while you prepare
the batter and sausages.

Crack the eggs into a jug, then whisk together with the flour
and a pinch of salt until smooth. Gradually whisk in the milk,
then set the batter aside to rest while you cook the sausages.

Heat 1 tablespoon of oil in a large frying pan over a medium
heat, then add the sausages and chopped rosemary and
cook, stirring, for 5 minutes until they have started to colour.
Remove the sausages from the pan and cut into halves.

Carefully remove the muffin tins from the oven, then pour
the Yorkshire pudding batter into the holes in the muffin
tins equally. Put half a chipolata into each muffin hole,
then return the pans to the oven and leave to cook for 15–20
minutes until the Yorkshire puddings are puffed and golden.

Meanwhile, return the pan that you cooked the sausages in
to the heat and add the onions along with the remaining
tablespoon of oil. Cook the onions, stirring occasionally, for
10 minutes until soft and golden, then add the peas,
vegetable bouillon powder and 2 tablespoons of flour. Stir
to coat the onions in the flour mixture, then gradually pour
in 600 ml/1 pint of boiling water, stirring and thickening
between each addition to form a gravy.

Divide the Yorkshire puddings between serving plates
(depending on appetites you may well have some left over
for another day), then spoon over the pea gravy. Serve with
steamed tenderstem broccoli on the side.

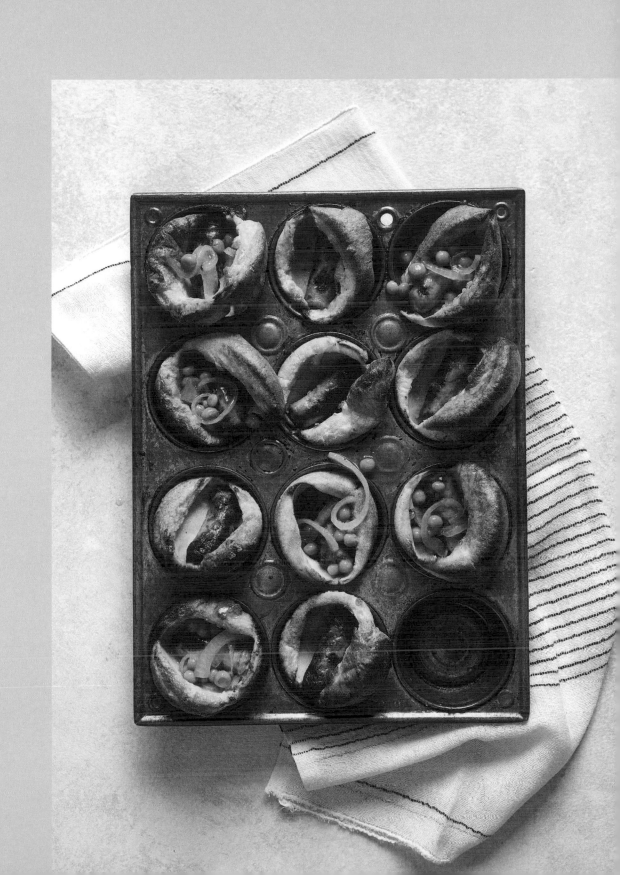

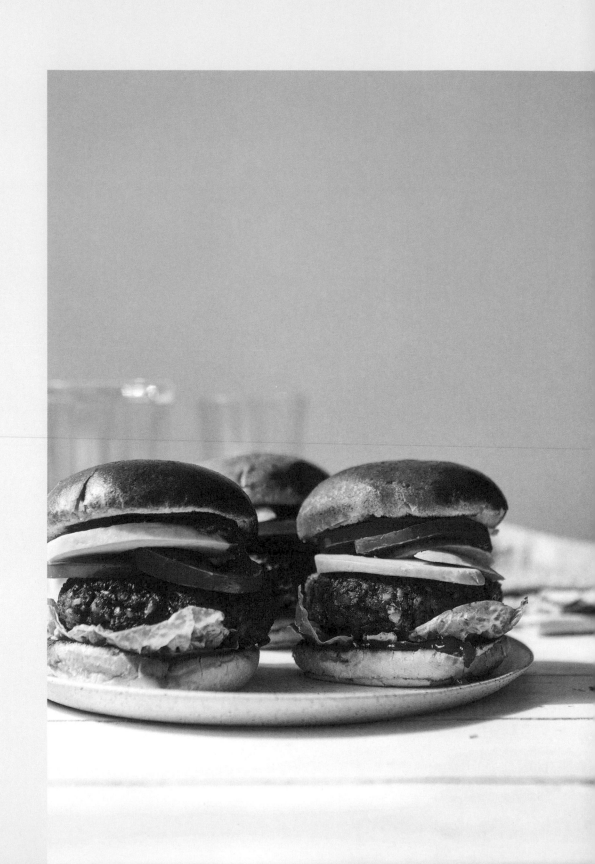

Veggie (or Beef) Burgers

After making these, you will never buy ready-made burgers again. So much better than any fast-food option, I make these burgers for both summer barbecues and family dinners. I've included both meat and veggie options. Alaia and I will always go for the veggie choice, whilst Marvin and Valle opt for the meat.

Prep: 15 minutes
Cook: 25 minutes
Makes 6

Put the onion and garlic in the bowl of a food processor and process until finely chopped (don't worry about washing up the food processor, as you will need it again later). Heat 1 tablespoon of the olive oil in a large frying pan over a medium heat, then add the chopped onion and garlic and cook, stirring occasionally, for 8–10 minutes until soft and golden. Tip the cooked onions and garlic into a large mixing bowl and set aside.

Put the kidney beans, beetroot and flour into the food processor (If you are making the veggie burgers, also add the peas and tofu to the food processor at this point) and process to a smooth paste. Add the bean and beetroot mixture to the bowl with the cooked onions. Rinse the bowl of the food processor, then add the porridge oats and 50 g/2 oz of the rice and pulse until combined, then tip this mixture into the bowl along with the remaining 50 g/2 oz of rice. (If you are making the beef burgers, add the minced beef to the bowl at this point.) Season generously, then, using your hands, give everything a mix until really well combined. Mould the mixture into 6 equal-sized patties, each around 10 cm/4 inches across and 1.5 cm/⅝ inch thick. Place in the fridge for at least 30 minutes to allow the burgers to firm up before cooking.

Heat the remaining tablespoon of oil in a large frying pan over a medium heat, then add the burgers and cook for 8–10 minutes on each side. (Depending on the size of your pan, you may need to do this in batches.) The burgers are quite delicate at first, so try not to move them around too much during cooking.

Once cooked, serve the burgers in brioche buns, topped with your choice of lettuce, sliced avocado, sliced tomato, mayonnaise and ketchup.

1 red onion, quartered
2 garlic cloves, peeled
2 tbsp olive oil
1 x 400 g/14 oz can kidney beans, drained
100 g/3½ oz cooked beetroot
100 g/3½ oz plain flour
2 tbsp porridge oats
100 g/3½ oz cooked brown rice (microwave pouches are ideal here)
sea salt and freshly ground black pepper
4 brioche buns, to serve
2 little gem lettuces, to serve
2 ripe avocados, peeled and sliced
2 large vine tomatoes, sliced
mayonnaise and ketchup, to serve

For the veggie burgers:
100 g/3½ oz frozen peas, defrosted
225 g/8 oz smoked firm tofu, drained

For the beef burgers:
400 g/14 oz minced beef

For first-stage weaning:
When babies are ready for finger foods, serve them chunks of burger and bun for grabbing.

For older children:
Omit the seasoning from the burger mix and serve with reduced-sugar ketchup, if desired.

Teriyaki Salmon

Prep: 5 minutes
Cook: 15 minutes
Serves 4

6 tbsp teriyaki sauce (check label for allergens)
juice of 1 lime
4 x 100 g/3½ oz skin-on salmon fillets
250 g/9 oz brown rice
200 g/7 oz fresh or frozen edamame beans
200 g/7 oz tenderstem broccoli
5 tsp sesame oil
¼ garlic clove, grated

For first-stage weaning:
Leave some of the salmon unmarinated, but cook in the same way, then mash the salmon into the cooked rice and serve with plain veg on the side.

For older children:
Older children should be fine with this as it is, though those with sensitive palates may prefer the veg served without the zingy dressing.

We are big salmon fans in my house and this dish is a firm favourite. The teriyaki marinade is zingy and delicious. Simply serve with brown rice and whatever greens you have in the fridge or freezer for a knock-out meal. I've suggested edamame beans, which I love as they are really versatile and packed with protein.

Put the teriyaki sauce and half of the lime juice in a wide, shallow bowl and mix to combine. Add the salmon fillets, skin-side up and set aside to marinate while you prepare the rice and veg.

Cook the rice in a pan of boiling water, according to packet instructions, until tender.

When the rice is almost ready, bring a pan of water to the boil over a high heat, the add the edamame beans and tenderstem broccoli, reduce to a simmer and leave to cook for 5 minutes until tender.

Heat 1 teaspoon of the sesame oil in a frying pan over a medium heat, then add the salmon, skin-side down, and half of the marinade. Cook for 5 minutes until the skin is crisp, then turn the salmon fillets and add the remaining marinade to the pan. Cook for another 3–5 minutes until the salmon is cooked through.

Meanwhile, combine the remaining lime juice, sesame oil and garlic in a small bowl and set aside.

Drain the rice and vegetables and divide between 4 serving bowls, then top each with a fillet of the salmon. Spoon the lime and sesame dressing over the vegetables in each bowl, then serve.

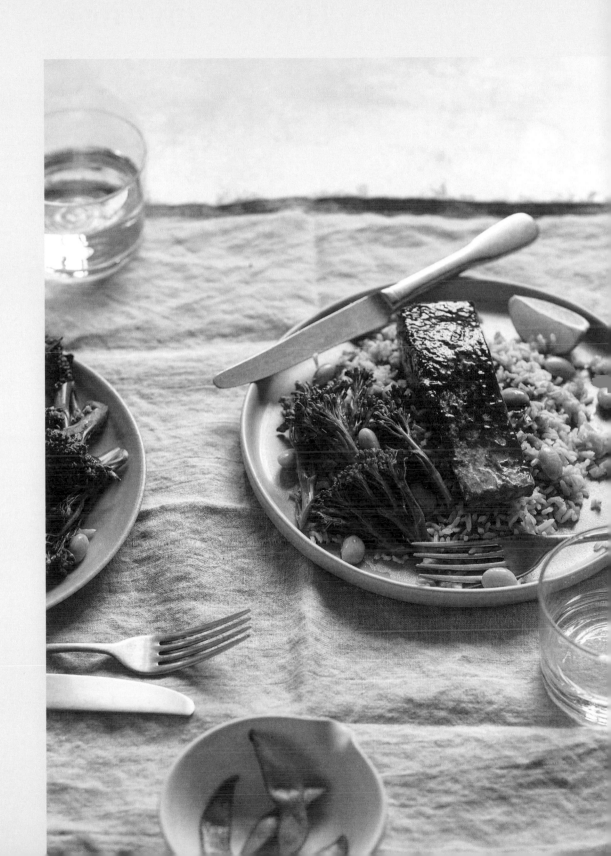

Thai Green Curry

Prep: 5 minutes
Cook: 20-25 minutes
Serves 4

1 tbsp vegetable oil
500 g/1 lb 2 oz skinless, boneless chicken thighs, cut into bite-sized pieces
1 aubergine, cut into 2 cm/¾ in pieces
1 yellow pepper, deseeded and finely sliced
2 tbsp good-quality Thai green curry paste (check label for allergens)
1 x 400 ml/14 fl oz can light coconut milk
200 g/7 oz green beans, trimmed and halved
cooked jasmine rice, to serve
lime wedges, to serve

For first-stage weaning:
The curry paste is too spicy and salty for very young palates, so fry of some of the chicken and vegetables separately, then blend to a purée with a little coconut milk or natural yoghurt. Serve with a small portion of rice alongside.

For older children:
Older children can enjoy this as it is, though you may want to serve with a dollop of natural yoghurt alongside for those sensitive to spice.

This deliciously fragrant curry is always a favourite, but takeaway versions can be expensive, so why not try making your own? I love the colour, spiciness, and texture of this curry. To save time, I always use shop-bought curry paste to make this and there are some really high-quality ones available in the shops.

Heat the oil in a large frying pan or wok over a medium heat, then add the chicken and aubergine and cook, stirring continuously, for 5 minutes, to seal the chicken. Add the sliced pepper to the pan along with the curry paste and 1 tablespoon of the coconut milk. Continue to cook for another 5 minutes, stirring occasionally until the pepper has softened and the paste is fragrant.

Add the remaining coconut milk to the pan and stir to combine. Bring the mixture to the boil, then reduce the heat to a simmer, cover with a lid and leave to cook for 5 minutes. Add the green beans to the curry and stir through, then cover again and cook for 5 minutes more until the chicken is cooked through and the vegetables are tender.

Spoon the curry into serving bowls and serve with jasmine rice alongside and lime wedges for squeezing over.

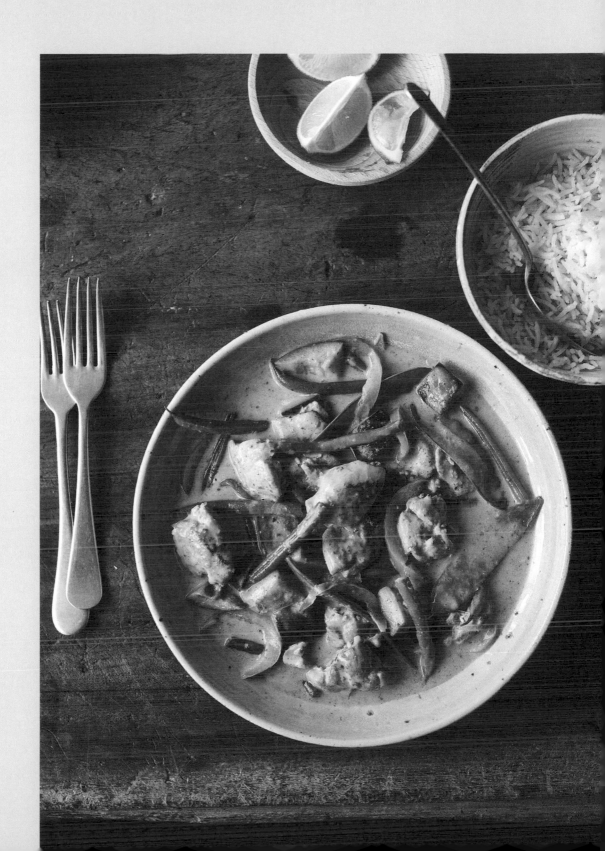

Family-Friendly Sunday Lunches

I know some people find cooking for large numbers a bit anxiety-provoking. I think if something is cooked with love then it will be fine! I always try and do a bit in advance, so I am never completely overwhelmed in the kitchen. Here are my favourite recipes for simple Sunday entertaining.

Lamb Rack with Mint Pesto

Prep: 5 minutes
Cook: 30 minutes
Serves 4

1 rack (between 6-8 cutlets) of French-trimmed lamb, caps, fat and sinews removed
1 garlic clove
small bunch basil, leaves picked
small bunch mint, leaves picked
25g/1 oz pine nuts (almonds or hazelnuts also work well)
25 g/1 oz Parmesan cheese, grated
125 ml/4 fl oz olive oil, plus 1 tbsp, for drizzling
juice of ½ lemon
sea salt and freshly ground pepper
cooked new potatoes and green beans, to serve

For first-stage weaning:
Children who are confident with finger foods will enjoy sucking the juices from a lamb cutlet.

For older children:
Older children will enjoy this dish as it is, but may need help to cut the lamb from the bone.

This is a delicious dish that is ideal for making for friends or dishing up to the family. The combination of tender lamb and fragrant mint pesto is incredible.

Preheat the oven to 200°C/400°F/gas mark 6.

To make the pesto, put the garlic, basil, mint, pine nuts and Parmesan into the bowl of a mini food processor or blender and blitz until well combined. Add the olive oil and lemon juice and blitz again to combine, then set aside while you prepare your lamb.

Drizzle the lamb racks with 1 tablespoon of olive oil and season generously all over, then rub a quarter of the pesto mixture into the lamb, using your hands to ensure it is well coated. Put a large griddle or frying pan over a medium heat and, once hot, add the lamb and sear for 2-3 minutes, turning the lamb with tongs until golden all over.

Transfer the lamb to a roasting tin and put in the oven to cook for 25 minutes. Once cooked, set the lamb aside to rest for 10 minutes, then slice into cutlets and serve with the rest of the pesto alongside. This is delicious served with buttery new potatoes and steamed green beans alongside.

Slow-Cooked Pork with Plum Sauce

This is a wonderful way of serving pork and makes a great dish for entertaining as you can get most of the cooking done before your guests arrive. After the long cooking time, the pork is wonderfully soft and sticky from the fragrant sauce. I have suggested serving this with rice and greens, but my kids also love this with mashed potato.

Preheat the oven to 140°C/275°F/gas mark 1.

Put the soy sauce, sriracha, tomato ketchup, hoisin, mirin, brown sugar and honey in a bowl, stir to combine and set aside.

Using a sharp knife, carefully slice the top layer of skin from the pork to expose the layer of fat. Score the fat at regular intervals all the way along the pork loin, slicing through the fat layer but not into the flesh. Rub the Chinese five spice all over the pork, then drizzle with 1 tablespoon of the sesame oil and rub that in also.

Put a roasting tin on the hob over a medium heat and add the remaining tablespoon of sesame oil. Once the oil is hot, add the shallots to the tin and cook, stirring continuously, for 2–3 minutes until starting to brown. Add the pork to the tin and cook for 5 minutes, turning occasionally with tongs until browned all over. Pour the sauce over the pork, then add the plums and chicken stock to the roasting tin and give everything a stir. Transfer the roasting tin to the oven and leave to cook for 4 hours, basting the pork in the sauce every hour until the meat is soft and falling-apart tender.

When the pork is almost cooked, bring 2 pans of water to the boil, then cook the rice and tenderstem broccoli until tender. Carve the pork and serve with the plum sauce from the tin spooned over and with rice and broccoli alongside.

Prep: 15 minutes
Cook: 4 hours
Serves 4

3½ tbsp soy sauce
1 tsp sriracha
3½ tbsp tomato ketchup (check label for allergens)
3½ tbsp hoisin sauce (check label for allergens)
3½ tbsp mirin
3½ tbsp brown sugar
3½ tbsp clear honey
1.25 kg/2 lb 12 oz pork loin
1½ tsp Chinese five spice
2 tbsp sesame oil
375 g/13 oz shallots, peeled and
6 ripe plums, halved and stoned
sea salt and freshly ground black pepper
250 ml/9 fl oz chicken stock
250 g/9 oz jasmine rice
500 g/1 lb 2 oz tenderstem broccoli

For first-stage weaning:
The sauce for is salty, sweet and spicy in equal measure, so is best avoided by children under 12 months. Simply serve them some of the rice and broccoli along with some shredded, uncoated meat from the centre of the loin.

For older children:
Adventurous older children will like this as it is, but serve the sauce moderately. Although there is some spice, the sauce is also sweet, so is a great way of introducing new flavours.

'Roch's Roasties' with Really Easy Roast Chicken, Broccoli & Brussels

Prep: 10 minutes
Cook: 1 hour 20 minutes
Serves 4

For 'Roch's Roasties':
1 kg/2 lb 4 oz Maris Piper potatoes
4 tbsp goose or duck fat
½ bunch thyme
sea salt and freshly ground black
    pepper

For the chicken and gravy:
4 sprigs rosemary, leaves picked
3 garlic cloves, peeled
2 tbsp olive oil
2 celery sticks, roughly chopped
2 carrots, peeled and roughly
    chopped
2 onions, roughly chopped
1.6 kg/3 lb 8 oz free-range chicken
2 tbsp plain flour
500 ml/18 fl oz chicken or vegetable
    stock
sea salt and freshly ground black
    pepper

For the brussels sprouts and broccoli:
450 g/1 lb brussels sprouts
1 tbsp olive oil
1 white onion, finely chopped
4 rashers smoked streaky bacon,
    finely sliced
1 star anise
½ tsp ground cinnamon
1 tbsp maple syrup
350 g/12 oz broccoli

When I first decided to write a cookbook one of the things that most spurred me on was my followers on social media asking for my recipes. And the recipe they asked for the most was my roast potatoes. Though for many the central focus of a roast is the meat, it's all about the potatoes in my house! I've highlighted the recipe for the roasties on their own below, as I know that some of you will want to make them without the suggested sides, but I've also suggested pairing them with roast chicken, broccoli and brussels sprouts if you want to make a full roast. Feel free to switch that up to suit your tastes and whatever veg are in season. Get the potatoes right and you can't go wrong!

Preheat the oven to 200°C/400°F/gas mark 6.

Grind the rosemary leaves and garlic together with a pestle and mortar, then add the olive oil and stir to combine.

Put the celery, carrots, and onions in the base of a large roasting tin and sit the chicken on top. Rub the chicken all over with the rosemary and garlic oil and season generously with salt and pepper. Transfer to the oven for 1 hour 10 minutes, basting hallway through the cooking time until the skin is crisp and golden and the flesh is juicy and cooked through. If the chicken is slightly smaller or larger, check the packet instructions and adjust the cooking time accordingly.

Once the chicken is in the oven, prepare the roast potatoes by following the recipe on the opposite page.

When the chicken is cooked, remove the tray from the oven and transfer the chicken to a carving tray. Cover with a couple of layers of foil, followed by a tea towel and set aside to allow the meat to rest while you finish up with the other elements. The chicken should be rested for at least 20 minutes and for up to an hour, so don't panic if it takes a while to get your other elements together.

Continued overleaf...

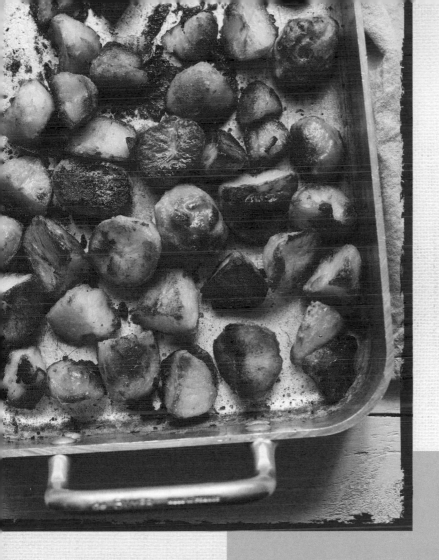

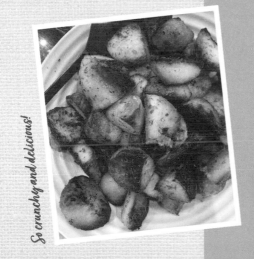

So crunchy and delicious!

FOR 'ROCH'S ROASTIES'

To make the roasties, put the potatoes in a large pan and cover with cold, salted water. Put over a high heat and bring just to the boil, then reduce the heat to a gentle simmer and leave to parboil for 8–10 minutes until starting to soften, but still firm in the centre. Drain through a colander and leave to steam fry for a couple of minutes.

Put another large, flameproof roasting tin on the hob over a medium heat and add the goose or duck fat. Once the fat has melted and is sizzling, carefully tip in the potatoes and turn them in the fat for a couple of minutes until they are starting to crisp and turn slightly golden. Add the thyme to the roasting tin and season the potatoes with salt and pepper, then carefully transfer the tin to the oven and roast the potatoes for 50 minutes until crisp and golden on the outside and soft and fluffy in the centre.

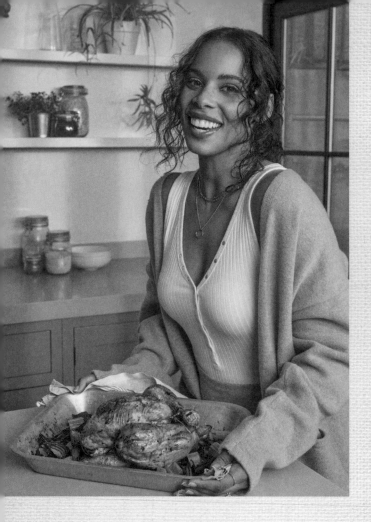

Put the roasting tin that the chicken was cooked in onto the hob over a medium-low heat. Using a potato masher, mash the roasted vegetables and fry them off in the chicken juices a little to give them a little colour, then add the flour and stir to a thick paste. Gradually pour in the chicken stock, stirring and thickening between each addition, then let the gravy bubble away for 10-15 minutes, while you prepare the vegetables.

Cut any larger brussels sprouts in half and remove and tatty outside leaves. Heat the olive oil in a frying pan, then add the sliced onion and bacon and cook, stirring continuously, for 2-4 minutes until golden. Add the star anise and ground cinnamon and stir to combine with the onions and bacon. Add the brussels sprouts to the pan along with a generous drizzle of maple syrup, then cook, stirring continuously, for around 5 minutes until the brussels are slightly golden and cooked through.

Steam or boil the broccoli for 5-10 minutes until tender. Strain the gravy through a sieve, pressing down to get as much flavour from the veg as possible, into jug or gravy boat. Carve the chicken. Put all the elements into serving dishes and place in the middle of the table for everyone to help themselves. Leave someone else to do the washing up!

For first-stage weaning
Add a couple of brussels sprouts to the pan with the broccoli when cooking, then purée the cooked veg with a little plain chicken breast. Due to the high salt content of the stock, young children should avoid the gravy. (Alternatively, use a reduced-salt stock when making the gravy.)

For older children:
Older children will enjoy this as it is. The potatoes can be very hot inside, so cut the kid's ones open to allow them to cool a little before serving.

One-Pot Roasted Salmon

I love a good one-pot meal and this recipe is one of my favourites. It is packed with Asian flavours, and I love the combination of sesame oil, garlic, lemon and ginger. Salmon is full of good fats, and is something I know my girls will always devour. Feel free to mix up the greens in this – if you don't have pak choi, just use broccoli, sugar snap peas or anything else green that you can get your hands on.

Preheat the oven to 180°C/350°F/gas mark 4.

To make the marinade, put the ginger, garlic, coriander stalks and a few leaves and a pinch of salt in a pestle and mortar or the bowl of a mini food processor and grind or process to a coarse paste. Add the soy sauce, 2 tablespoons of the sesame oil and the juice of half the lemon, then grind or process again to combine.

Put the salmon, skin-side up, in a shallow bowl, then pour over the marinade and set aside to marinate while you prepare the potatoes.

Put the potatoes in a large pan and cover with cold, salted water, cutting any larger potatoes into halves as you do. Place over a high heat and bring just to the boil, then lower the heat to a simmer and leave to cook for 5 minutes. Add your chosen greens to the pan and leave to cook for another 3 minutes, then drain the potatoes and veg through a colander and leave to steam dry for a couple of minutes.

Tip the potatoes and greens into a roasting tin in an even layer, then place the salmon, skin-side down, over the top. Pour the marinade over the dish and drizzle with the remaining tablespoon of olive oil. Cut the remaining half lemon into wedges and add those to the tin, too, then transfer to the oven and cook for 20–25 minutes until the salmon is cooked through and the potatoes are crisp and tender.

Pick the baked lemon wedges from the tin and squeeze over the salmon, then discard. Divide the salmon and vegetables between serving plates and top with a scattering of coriander leaves. Serve hot.

Prep: 10 minutes
Cook: 25 minutes
Serves 4

35 g/1¼ oz fresh ginger, peeled and roughly chopped
3 garlic cloves
1 bunch coriander, leaves picked and stalks chopped
2 tbsp soy sauce
3 tbsp sesame oil
1 lemon
4 x 100 g/3½ skin-on salmon fillets
600 g/1 lb 5 oz new potatoes
300 g/10½ oz greens (pak choi, broccoli, asparagus, etc.)
sea salt and freshly ground black pepper

For first-stage weaning:
Cook a portion of the salmon and vegetables in a separate tray without the marinade, then purée the cooked salmon and veg. Always check fish for bones before serving to children.

For older children:
Older children can enjoy this at it is, just be sure to check the salmon for any bones before serving and use a reduced-salt soy sauce when making the marinade.

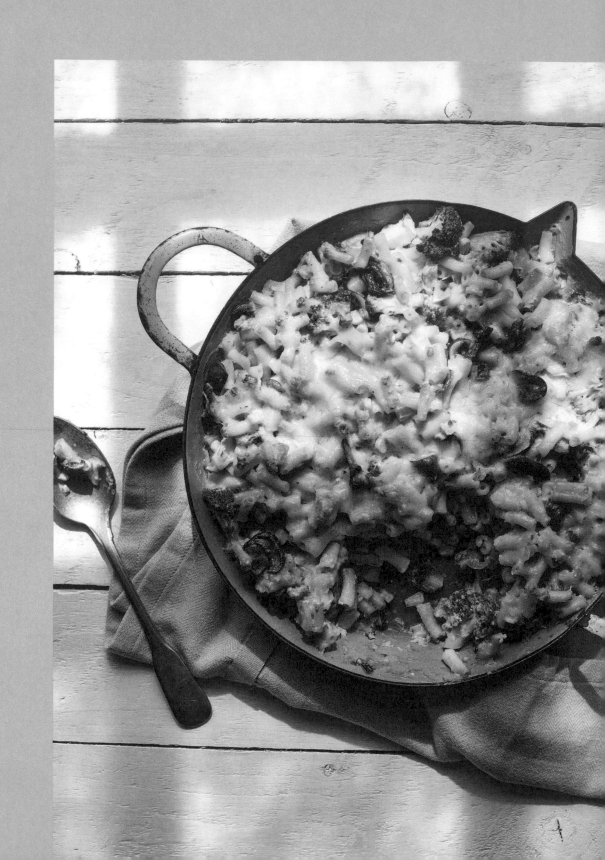

Ultimate Mac & Cheese

Give your mac & cheese a kid-friendly upgrade by adding loads of veg to it. It still feels like a treat, so I know my kids will eat it, but it is also packed with good stuff. I often add broccoli, red onions and mushrooms, but other veg like peas and cauliflower will also taste great, so throw in whatever you have to use up.

If you would like to bake the macaroni cheese, preheat the oven to 200°C/400°F/gas mark 6.

Bring a large pan of salted water to the boil over a medium heat, add the macaroni and cook for 5–10 minutes, according to packet instructions until tender. Strain the macaroni, reserving a mugful of the pasta water.

While the pasta is cooking, prepare the sauce. Heat the oil in a large pan over a medium heat, then add the red onion and mushroom, and cook, stirring occasionally, for 8–10 minutes until soft and golden.

Add the butter to the pan and, once melted, add the flour and cook, stirring continuously, for 1–2 minutes to make a thick paste. Add a little of the milk and stir into the flour mixture until thickened, then keep adding the milk in stages, stirring and thickening between each addition until you have a thick, glossy sauce. Add the grated cheese and broccoli, and cook, stirring occasionally, for 5 minutes until the broccoli is tender. If you are serving this to vegetable-averse children, you can blend the sauce with a stick blender at this stage until smooth.

Add the sweetcorn to the pan, draining it if using canned, and stir to combine, then tip in the cooked pasta and reserved pasta water and stir again. Season to taste.

The macaroni cheese could now be spooned into serving bowls and served, but to make it extra special I often transfer it to a baking dish, scatter with a little extra grated cheese and bake for 25–30 minutes until golden and bubbling. Any leftovers can be left to cool, then stored in the fridge or freezer for another day.

Prep: 15 minutes
Cook: 20–45 minutes
Serves 4 (with leftovers for another day)

300 g/10½ oz dried macaroni
1 tbsp olive oil
1 red onion, finely chopped
150 g/5 oz mushrooms, halved and sliced
15 g/½ oz unsalted butter
2 tbsp plain flour
850 ml/1½ pints whole milk (or dairy-free alternative)
100 g/3½ oz mature Cheddar cheese, grated, plus extra if baking
160 g/5¾ oz broccoli, stems finely sliced and florets cut into bite-sized pieces
200 g/7 oz frozen or canned sweetcorn
sea salt and freshly ground black pepper

For first-stage weaning:
Make the macaroni cheese without any seasoning, then blitz a small portion to a purée. You could also stir through some cooked peas and small pieces of cooked cauliflower to introduce a bit of texture.

For older children:
Older children will enjoy the macaroni cheese at it is, just pass salt and pepper around to the adults separately when serving.

One-Pot Veggie, Bean & Quinoa Stew

Prep: 10 minutes
Cook: 30 minutes
Serves 4

100 g/3½ oz quinoa
1 tbsp olive oil
1 onion, finely chopped
1 garlic clove, crushed
1 leek, trimmed and finely chopped
1½ tsp ground cinnamon
2 x 400g/14 oz cans chopped
  tomatoes
850 ml/1½ pints vegetable stock
1 carrot, peeled and cut into 2 cm/
  ¾ in pieces
250 g/9 oz broccoli, cut into small
  florets
150 g/5 oz cabbage, shredded
  (sweetheart, white and savoy all
  work well)
1 x 400g/14 oz can kidney beans,
  drained
1 x 400g/14 oz can cannellini or other
  white beans, drained
handful of grated Parmesan cheese,
  to serve
sea salt and freshly ground black
  pepper

This one-pot wonder is really versatile and great for using up veggies that are on the turn. When one of the kids has a cold, I add all the veggies I can get my hands on for extra vitamins. If there are leftovers, I will eat it the next day for lunch with mashed potato or brown rice. Alternatively, you can freeze some for a later date. Sometimes, for variety, I will add dumplings.

Put the quinoa in a sieve and rinse under cold running water until the water runs clear. Set aside.

Heat the oil in a large pan over a medium heat, then add the onion, garlic and leek and fry, stirring continuously, for 5 minutes until softened. Stir through the cinnamon, then tip in the chopped tomatoes and vegetable stock and stir again to combine.

Add the carrot, broccoli, cabbage and both types of bean to the pan, along with the quinoa. Bring the mixture to the boil, then reduce to a simmer and leave to cook, stirring occasionally, for 20 minutes until the quinoa has swelled and all of the vegetables are tender. Season the stew to taste, then ladle into a serving bowl and garnish with a little grated Parmesan. Serve hot.

For first-stage weaning:
Make the stew with reduced-salt stock and omit the seasoning, then blend a small portion to a purée for any very young children.

For older children:
Older children can enjoy this as it is, just leave out the seasoning and pass it around separately to the adults when serving the meal. For any children who are fussy with texture, you could blend a portion of the stew and serve it as a sauce over cooked pasta.

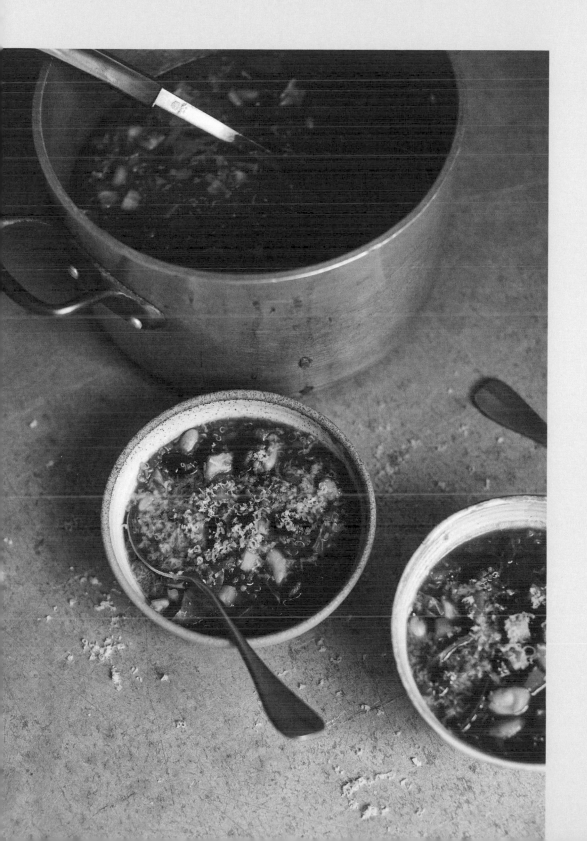

Pork Ramen Noodle Soup

Prep: 5 minutes
Cook: 30 minutes
Serves 4

2 tbsp sesame oil
200 g/7 oz minced pork
2 garlic cloves, finely sliced
2 thumb-sized pieces ginger, peeled and cut into matchsticks
½ tsp Chinese five spice
2 tbsp soy sauce
1 bunch spring onions, white and green parts finely sliced
400 g/14 oz medium egg noodles
2 large eggs
1-2 star anise
2 litres/3½ pints chicken or vegetable stock
4 pak choi, halved
sea salt and freshly ground black pepper

For first-stage weaning:
The soy in this is too salty for very young children, but they can have some chopped hard-boiled egg, which you could purée with some of the noodles and cooked vegetables.

For older children:
Older children can enjoy this as it is, just use a reduced-salt soy sauce when preparing the ramen.

Bring your favourite Japanese restaurant home with this pork ramen recipe. The best family dinners are full of flavour, nutritious and super-simple to prepare, and this ticks all of those boxes! It is also light, but really warming and comforting. My kids love eating with chopsticks, so we always have a few pairs in the house – just be prepared to clear up the mess afterwards!

Heat 1 tablespoon of the oil in a large pan over a medium heat. Add the pork mince, garlic, ginger, Chinese five spice, soy sauce and white parts of the spring onions and cook, stirring continuously, for 5 minutes until the meat has browned and is starting to caramelize. Tip the spiced pork mixture into a bowl and keep it warm while you prepare the other elements.

Bring a pan of water the boil and add the eggs and noodles. Cook for 6 minutes, then drain the noodles and set aside. Rinse the eggs under cold water for a couple of minutes, then peel off and discard the shells and cut the eggs into halves.

Meanwhile, return the pan that the pork was cooked in to the heat with the remaining tablespoon of sesame oil. Add the star anise to the pan and fry briefly until fragrant, then pour in the chicken or vegetable stock. Bring the mixture to the boil, then reduce to a simmer and add the pak choi. Leave to cook for 4 minutes until the pak choi is tender.

To serve the ramen, divide the broth, noodles, pork and egg halves between 4 serving bowls. Scatter over the green parts of the spring onions and serve hot.

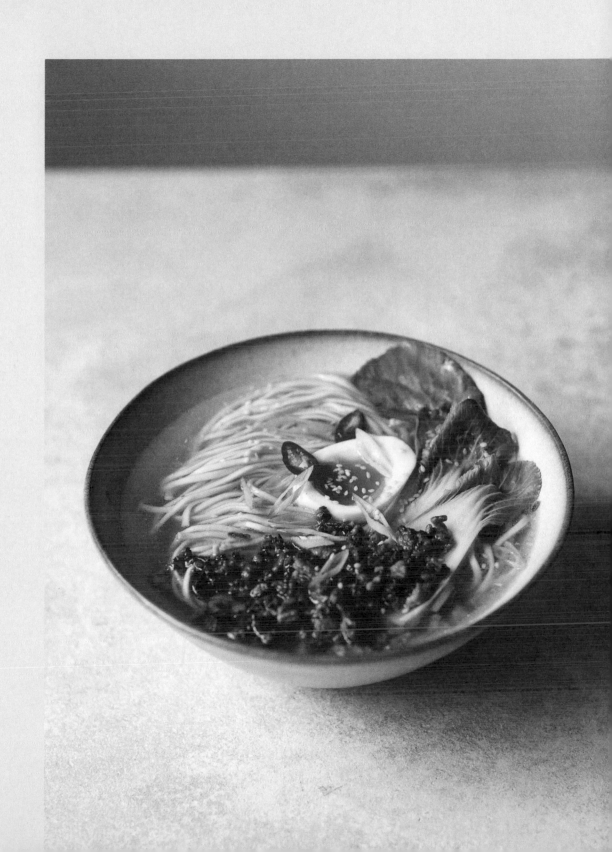

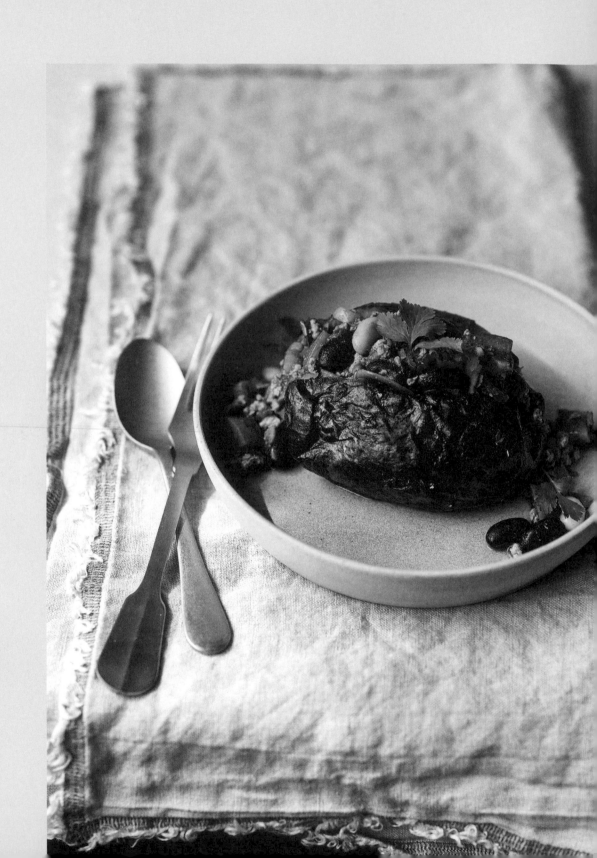

Sweet Turkey Chilli

Turkey brings some variety to the table, plus it is lean, low-fat and budget-friendly. If you ever fancy a change from minced beef for other recipes, then try subbing in turkey. This recipe can be served with jacket potatoes, or brown rice and a crunchy salad.

Heat the oil in a large pan over a medium heat, then add the onion, carrot, celery, courgette, garlic, stalks from the coriander and smoked paprika and stir to combine. Fry the vegetables for 10 minutes, stirring continuously until softened and starting to caramelize.

Add the minced turkey to the pan and continue to cook for 5 minutes, stirring to break down the mince with a wooden spoon until browned. Add the chopped tomatoes, then carefully fill the can with boiling water and tip that in also. Tip in both types of beans and stir the mixture to combine. Bring the chilli to the boil, then reduce to a simmer, cover with a lid, and leave to cook for 20 minutes, removing the lid for the last 5 minutes of the cooking time.

Season the chilli to taste, then stir through the coriander leaves, spoon into serving bowls and serve with your choice of accompaniments.

Prep: 5 minutes
Cook: 40-45 minutes
Serves 4

1 tbsp olive oil
1 onion, halved and finely sliced
1 carrot, peeled and finely chopped
2 celery sticks, finely chopped
1 courgette, trimmed and finely chopped
2 garlic cloves, crushed
1 small bunch coriander, leaves picked and stalks finely chopped
1 heaped tsp smoked paprika
500 g/1 lb 2 oz minced turkey
1 x 400 g/14 oz can chopped tomatoes
1 x 400 g/14 oz can kidney beans, drained
1 x 400 g/14 oz can cannellini beans, drained
sea salt and freshly ground black pepper
jacket potatoes, brown rice or crunch salad, to serve

For first-stage weaning:
Blitz a small portion of the chilli to a purée and serve with some rice on the side.

For older children:
The spicing in this is delicate, so this can easily be enjoyed as it is by children of all ages.

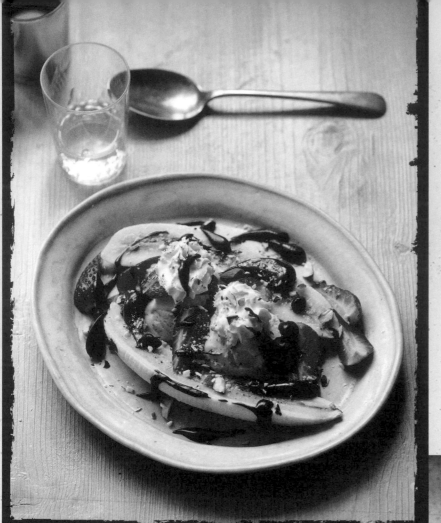

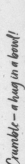

Crumble — a hug in a bowl!

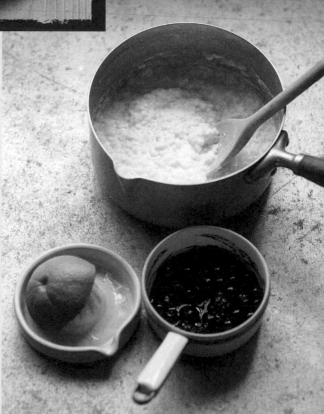

Pudding is my absolute favourite part of any meal. When I'm in a restaurant, I'll always look at the pudding menu before making any decision about my main course! Whether it is an everyday treat or something more decadent for a dinner party, my puddings cover all the bases. You'll find my best pudding recipes here, from classic favourites like Banana Split (see page 174) to Peach Melba Pancakes (see page 179).

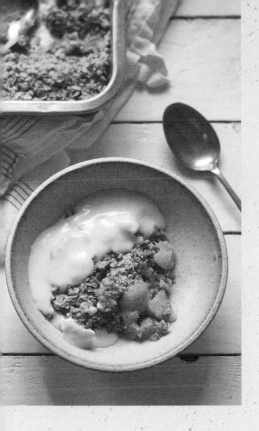

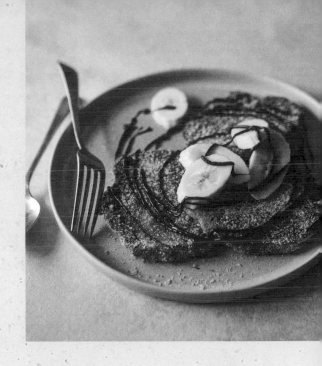

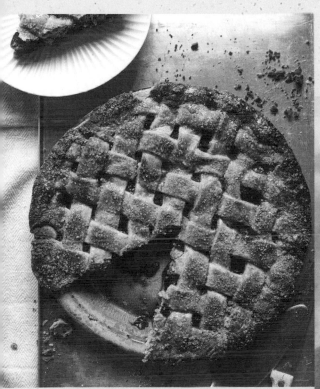

Puddings

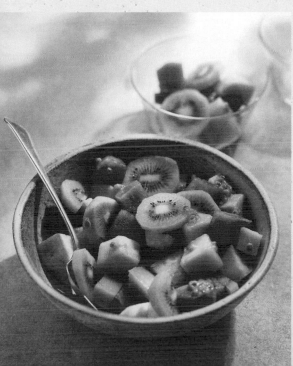

Cake Pops

Prep: 15 minutes, plus cooling
   and setting
Cook: 20 minutes
Makes 15

125 g/4½ oz butter
150 g/5 oz caster sugar
2 large eggs
150 g/5 oz self-raising flour
For the buttercream icing:
100 g/3½ oz unsalted butter,
   softened to room temperature
150 g/5½ oz icing sugar
50 g/1¾ oz cocoa powder
2 tbsp milk
300 g/10½ oz milk chocolate,
   broken into small chunks
50 g/1¾ sprinkles or edible glitter

For first-stage weaning:
These treats aren't suitable
for very young children.

For older children:
These are great occasional
treats for older children, who will
enjoy making them almost as
much as eating them! They
make wonderful party-bag
treats for a children's party.

Cake pops are fantastic for kids' parties and special occasions when you want to end with something sweet, but don't want a large wedge of cake or a full-on dessert. They look so pretty and can be decorated in any way you like, which the kids will love helping with. You may think these look a bit fiddly, but I promise that they are much easier than they look.

Preheat the oven to 190°C/375°F/gas mark 5 and grease a square 20-cm/8-inch cake pan with butter and line with greaseproof paper. Line a baking sheet with greaseproof paper.

Using a stand mixer or electric whisk, beat the butter and sugar together for 5 minutes until light and fluffy. Crack the eggs into the mixture one at a time, beating to incorporate between each addition, then sift in the flour and fold into the mixture until well combined.

Pour the mixture into the prepared cake tin and level out with a spatula. Transfer to the oven and bake for 20 minutes until golden, well risen and an inserted skewer comes out clean. Leave to cool in the tin for 10 minutes, then turn out onto a wire rack and leave to cool to room temperature.

While the cake is cooling, make the buttercream icing. Using a stand mixer or electric whisk, beat together the butter, icing sugar, cocoa powder and milk for 5 minutes until smooth.

Once the cake has cooled, crumble the sponge into the bowl with the buttercream, then stir the mixture to make sure everything is well combined. Using your hands, roll the mixture into 15 golf ball-sized balls, insert a lolly stick into each one and lay them flat on the prepared baking sheet. Transfer to the fridge for an hour to firm up.

Continued overleaf...

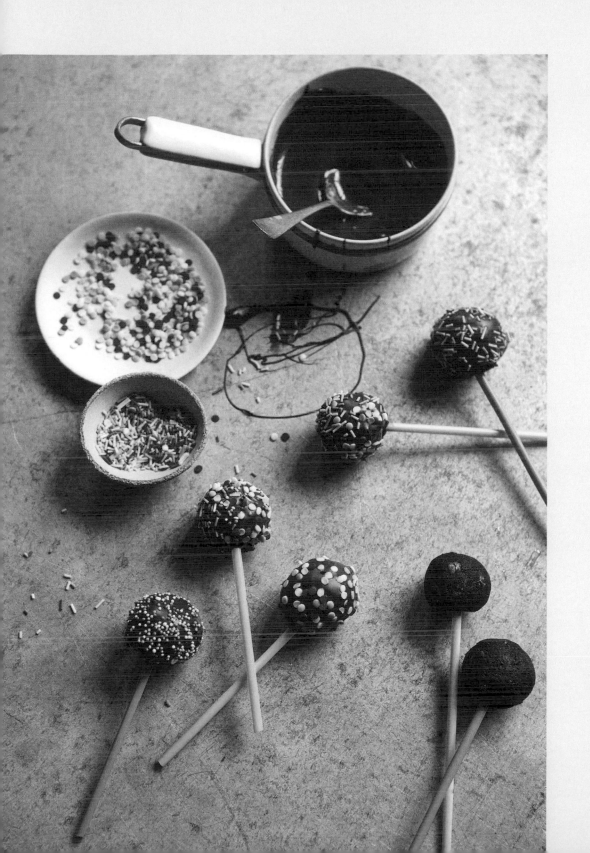

While the cake pops are setting, melt the chocolate either in the microwave in short bursts or in a heatproof bowl set over a pan of simmering water. Put the sprinkles or edible glitter in a bowl on the counter and set the bowl of melted chocolate next to it.

Working quickly, dip one of the cake pops into the melted chocolate, completely submerging the end of the pop so that it is fully coated in chocolate, let any melted chocolate drip off, then immediately roll the chocolate-coated pop in the sprinkles or edible glitter. Stand the coated cake pop in a cup or jar while you repeat the process with the remaining cake pops.

Once all of the cake pops are coated, leave to set at room temperature for 30 minutes, then transfer to the fridge for a further hour to fully firm up. These will keep in the fridge for a few days.

Cherry Pie

This sweet, summery dessert is so wonderful dished up with cream or vanilla ice cream. It is one dessert in my family that no one ever wants to miss, especially Marvin. He is a not a dessert person, but he goes mad for this. The lattice on top may look intimidating, but is actually surprisingly easy and looks really impressive!

Tip one of the cans of cherries into a pan. Place a sieve or colander over a bowl and strain the second can of cherries through it, reserving the syrup. Put the strained cherries into the pan, then mix 2 tablespoons of cornflour with 2 tablespoons of the reserved cherry liquid and add that to the pan also, along with the cinnamon, vanilla extract and orange zest. Put the pan over a medium heat and bring to the boil, then reduce to a simmer and leave to cook, stirring occasionally, for 5 minutes until thickened. Remove from the heat and leave to cool to room temperature, while you make the pastry.

Put the butter, icing sugar, flour and egg yolks in the bowl of a food processor, then pulse until the mixture resembles breadcrumbs. Add 1 tablespoon of the milk and pulse again until the mixture just comes together into a ball, adding the remaining milk if necessary. Form the mixture into a ball, wrap in plastic film or greaseproof paper and transfer to the fridge to rest for 30 minutes.

While the pastry is resting, preheat the oven to 200°C/400°F/gas mark 6 and grease a 23 cm/9 inch pie dish with butter.

Slice the pastry into 2 pieces, one slightly larger than the other, and return the smaller piece to the fridge. Roll the larger piece of the pastry out on a lightly floured surface until it is 3 mm/⅛ inch thick (around the thickness of a £1 coin) and large enough to line the base of your pie dish. Using the rolling pin to lift it, lay the pastry over the base of the pie dish, allowing any excess to hang over the edge.

Prep: 40 minutes, plus resting and cooling
Cook: 30–35 minutes
Serves 6

2 x 400g/14 oz cans cherries in syrup
2 tbsp cornflour
1 cinnamon stick
1 tsp vanilla extract
zest of 1 orange
custard, cream or ice cream, to serve

For the pastry:
125 g/4½ oz cold unsalted butter, cut into cubes
100 g/3½ oz icing sugar
250 g/9 oz plain flour
2 egg yolks
1–2 tbsp milk, plus extra for brushing
1 tbsp granulated or demerara sugar

Continued overleaf...

For first-stage weaning:
This is too sweet for children under 12 months. For older babies and toddlers, you could blitz a tablespoon of the tinned cherries with a little yoghurt to a sweet purée for an occasional treat.

For older children:
Older kids will love this pie as it is.

Remove and discard the cinnamon stick from the cooled pie filling, then pour the filling into the pie. Remove the other half of the pastry from the fridge and roll it out in the same way, then use a sharp knife or pizza cutter to slice it into 10 long strips, each approximately 2 cm/¾ inch wide. Lay a sheet of greaseproof paper on the work top and arrange 5 pastry strips horizontally on it. Now weave the other 5 strips of pastry vertically over and under the horizontal strips to create a lattice. Carefully slide the lattice onto the top of the pie, and tuck and crimp with the bottom layer of pastry at the edges to seal. Trim any excess pastry, then brush the top with a little milk and sprinkle over the sugar.

Transfer the pie to the oven to bake for 25–30 minutes until the pastry is golden brown and the filling is bubbling. Set aside for 30 minutes, to allow the filling to cool and set slightly, then cut into slices and serve with custard, cream, ice cream, or a combination of the lot!

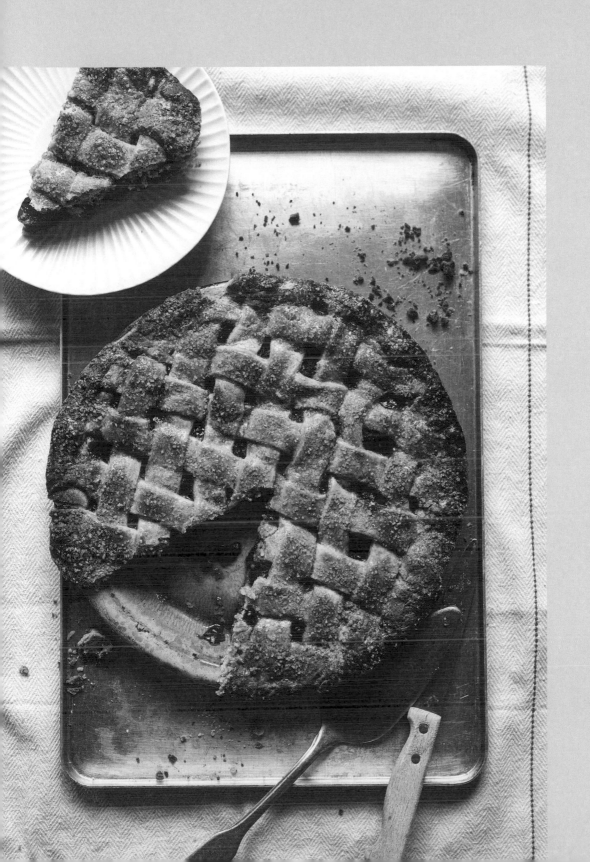

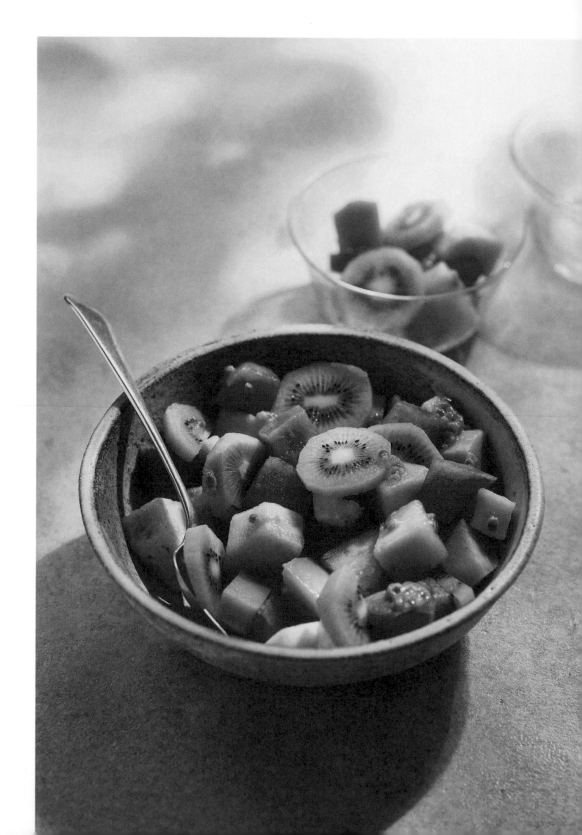

Tropical Fruit Salad

My kids devour all fruit, so they absolutely love this tropical salad, which feels a lot more special and celebratory than simply grabbing an apple from the fruit bowl! It is so colourful and refreshing, and you can pop other fruit you have at home in it too. I have put it in the pudding section, but it is great at any time of the day, especially at breakfast.

Put the prepared mango, pineapple, melon or watermelon and kiwi into a large bowl and give everything a good mix to combine. Scoop out the pulp from the passion fruits and add to the bowl, then mix again. Put the bowl in the middle of the table and let everyone dig in.

Prep: 10 minutes
Serves 4

1 ripe mango, halved, peeled and chopped into bite-size pieced
300 g/10½ oz pineapple, peeled and cut into 2 cm/¾ in thick fingers
200 g/7 oz melon or watermelon, rind removed and flesh cut into bite-sized pieces
2 kiwis, peeled and sliced or cut into bite-sized pieces
2 passion fruit, halved

First-stage weaning:
Cut the fruit into larger fingers to make it easy for very young children to explore it with their hands and mouths. If you are just starting out on weaning, introduce foods one at a time so that you can safely check for any allergies.

For older children:
This makes a wonderful, healthy dessert for older children. Just ensure that the fruit is chopped small enough not to pose a choking hazard.

Food Experiments You Can Eat

Food games can be really fun! Earlier in the book (see pages 34-5), I mentioned that there are loads of benefits to playing with food for little ones and I've found that as my girls have got older, there are more and more fun games that we can have with food. Here are some fun ideas to get started.

Build a Tower

What do you need?
· grapes, cucumber slices, strawberries, or marshmallows
· cocktail sticks (for older kids)

Get your kids to use the food to make a tower. Younger children will enjoy stacking cucumber or marshmallows to see how high they can make it. This a great for hand/eye coordination. Older children can use cocktail sticks to make weird and wonderful constructions and towers. Tell them to keep building until it falls down!

Chopstick Challenge

What do you need?
· a set of chopsticks for each child
· Maltesers, Smarties, small pieces of chopped fruit

This is another fun game for older kids, or a great kids' party game. Give each child (or team) two bowls. Fill one with Maltesers, Smarties or small pieces of fruit. Set the timer for 1 minute and see how many of the food items they can get from one bowl to the other using the chopsticks. When the game is finished, everyone gets to eat the treats!

Blindfold Taste Test

What do you need?
· mixed fruit and berries, chopped into bite-sized pieces
· a blindfold

Time for a taste test! Blindfold the children and get them to taste and guess the different fruity flavours. This is really fun and the whole family can join in.

Tray-Baked Plums or Peaches

Some of the best recipes are surprisingly easy. This is a lovely treat dessert for the kids and a great way to satisfy everyone's sweet cravings, whilst also serving something nutritious. You can use either plums or peaches with this, so make it with whatever is in season. It also tastes amazing the day after for breakfast.

Preheat the oven to 180°C/350°F/gas mark 4.

Lay the plums or peaches, cut-side up in a baking dish, then pour over the apple juice and sprinkle over the sugar, ensuring that each plum or peach half gets a little sprinkling. Add the cinnamon stick to the dish, then cover with foil and transfer to the oven for 40 minutes until the fruit is soft and fragrant.

Divide the cooked fruit between serving bowls and spoon a generous dollop of yoghurt into each one. Serve while the fruit is still hot.

Prep: 5 minutes
Cook: 40 minutes
Serves 4

6 ripe plums or peaches, halved
  and stones removed
125 ml/4 fl oz apple juice
2 tbsp sugar
1 cinnamon stick
500 g/1 lb 2 oz Greek yoghurt

For first-stage weaning:
Omit the sugar when baking the fruit, then mash some of the cooked fruit and serve with a spoonful of yoghurt alongside.

For older children:
Older children will enjoy this as it is.

Apple Crumble

Prep: 5 minutes
Cook: 30-40 minutes
Serves 4-6

4 cooking apples (approx. 700 g/
   1 lb 9 oz), peeled, cored and cut
   into 3 cm/1¼ in chunks
175 ml/6 fl oz apple juice
200 g/7 oz cold unsalted butter, cut
   into cubes
200 g/7 oz plain flour
1 tsp ground ginger
100 g/3½ oz golden caster sugar
200 g/7 oz porridge oats
custard or ice cream, to serve

For first-stage weaning:
Blitz some of the cooked apples
to a purée and fold through some
plain yoghurt.

For older children:
Older children will love this as
it is and can get involved in the
kitchen by helping to make the
crumble. If you are worried about
sugar, serve the crumble with
yoghurt rather than ice cream
or custard.

You can't beat a traditional apple crumble for dessert.
This all-time autumn and winter favourite has a lovely
crumbly top with soft, sweet apples in the middle.
Warming and comforting, this is the perfect finish to
a family weekend meal.

Preheat the oven to 180°C/350°F/gas mark 4.

Put the apples and apple juice in a pan over a medium heat,
bring to the boil, then reduce the heat to a simmer and cook,
stirring occasionally, for 2-3 minutes until the apples have
started to soften but still retain some bite. Tip the apples
into a large baking dish and set side while you prepare the
crumble.

Put the butter, flour and ginger in a large mixing bowl. Using
your hands, rub the butter into the flour until the mixture
resembles breadcrumbs, then add the sugar and porridge
oats and give the mixture a stir to combine.

Spoon the crumble over the apple in the dish in an even
layer, then transfer the crumble to the oven to cook for
35-40 minutes until golden and bubbling. Leave to cool
for 5 minutes, then spoon into serving bowls and serve with
custard or ice cream alongside.

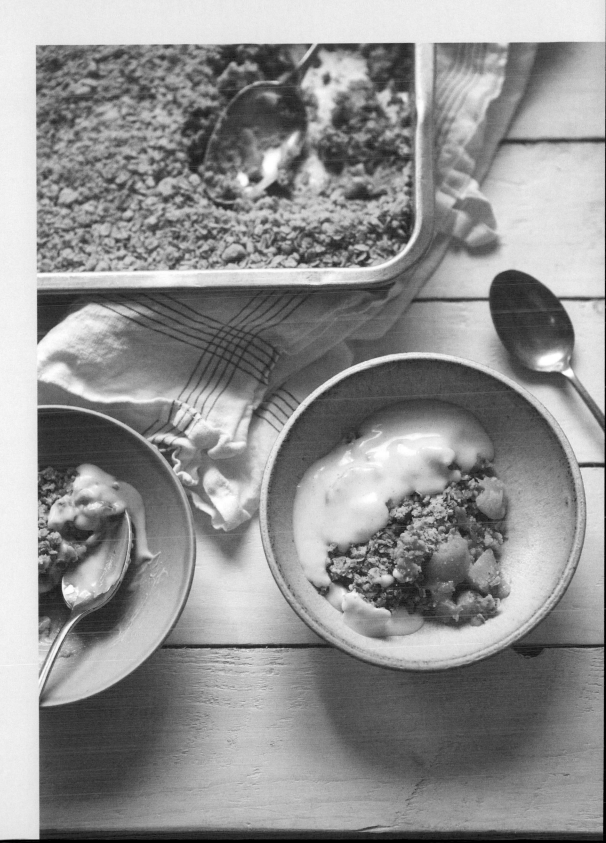

Fruity Fool

Prep: 10 minutes
Cook: 5 minutes
Serves 4

150 g/5 oz raspberries
2 tbsp elderflower cordial
100 ml/3½ fl oz double cream
100 g/3½ oz Greek yoghurt
handful of toasted coconut flakes

For first-stage weaning.
Make very young babies their own bowl with just some raspberries and yoghurt.

For older children:
Allergies permitting, older children can enjoy the fools as they are.

Fruit fool is such a simple idea, but one that is always a hit with the smallest members of the family. You can make it using whatever fruit you have to hand. It is great with berries and other sweet or tangy fruits that cut through the creamy yoghurt.

Put the raspberries and elderflower cordial in a pan over a medium heat. Bring to the boil, then reduce the heat to a simmer and leave to cook for 5 minutes until the raspberries are soft and pulpy. Set the mixture aside until cooled to room temperature.

Once cooled, spoon a quarter of the cooked raspberries into a small bowl and set aside. Put the remaining raspberries in the jug of a blender and blitz until smooth.

Put the cream in a large bowl and whip with an electric whisk until soft peaks form. Fold the yoghurt and blended raspberries through the cream, then divide the mixture between 4 serving bowls or glasses. Transfer the fools to the fridge for 2 hours to firm up.

Once firm, remove the fools from the fridge and spoon the reserved cooked raspberries over the top. Scatter over the toasted coconut flakes and serve

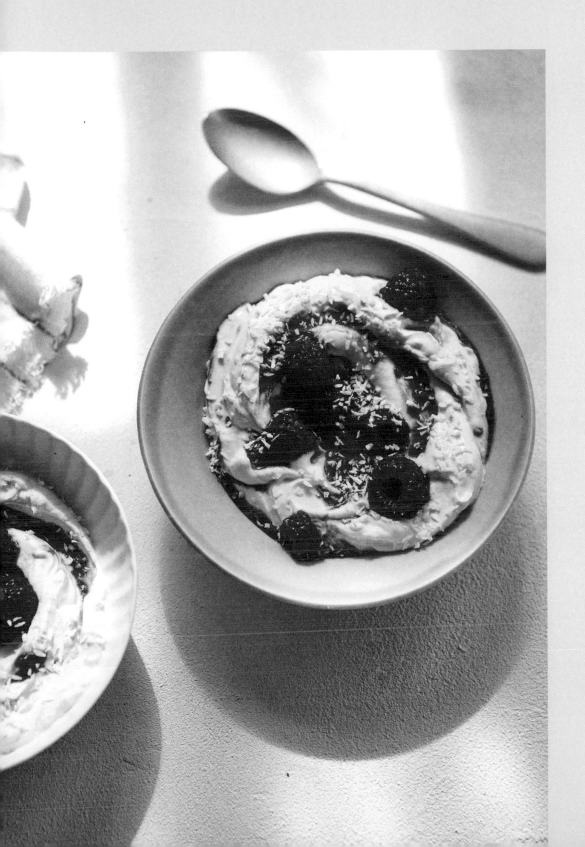

Banana Split

Prep: 5 minutes
Cook: 2 minutes
Serves 4

15 g/½ oz whole almonds
3–4 ripe bananas
250 g/9 oz strawberries, hulled
  and quartered
4–8 scoops good-quality vanilla
  ice cream
squirty cream (optional)

For the sauce:
100 g/3½ oz 70% dark chocolate,
  broken into chunks
30 g/1 oz unsalted butter
85 ml/3 fl oz semi-skimmed milk

For first-stage weaning:
Cut some banana into large
chunks and serve with some of
the quartered strawberries.

For older children:
Cut the strawberries into smaller
pieces to avoid any chance of
choking. Serve with yoghurt
rather than ice cream and cream,
or serve the dish as it is for an
occasional treat.

This is my take on a classic split, made with bananas,
vanilla ice cream, strawberries, cream, dark chocolate
and peanuts, and it always gets a thumbs up from
everyone. You can tweak the toppings or add any
flavour ice cream as you like. It is one of our weekend
favourites and really yummy.

First, make the sauce by heating the chocolate and butter
over a low heat until melted. Stir through the milk until the
sauce is well combined and glossy, then remove from the
heat and set aside while you prepare the other elements.

Put a small frying pan over a medium heat, add the whole
almonds and cook, moving the nuts in the pan continuously
to prevent them catching until toasted. Tip onto a chopping
board and roughly chop, then set aside.

Peel the bananas and slice into long halves. Divide the
bananas between serving dishes, giving 2 halves to adults
and 1 half to any children. Spoon the strawberries around the
bananas, then add 1–2 scoops of vanilla ice cream to each
plate. Add a couple of squirts of cream to each serving, if
using, then drizzle over the chocolate sauce and scatter over
the chopped, toasted almonds.

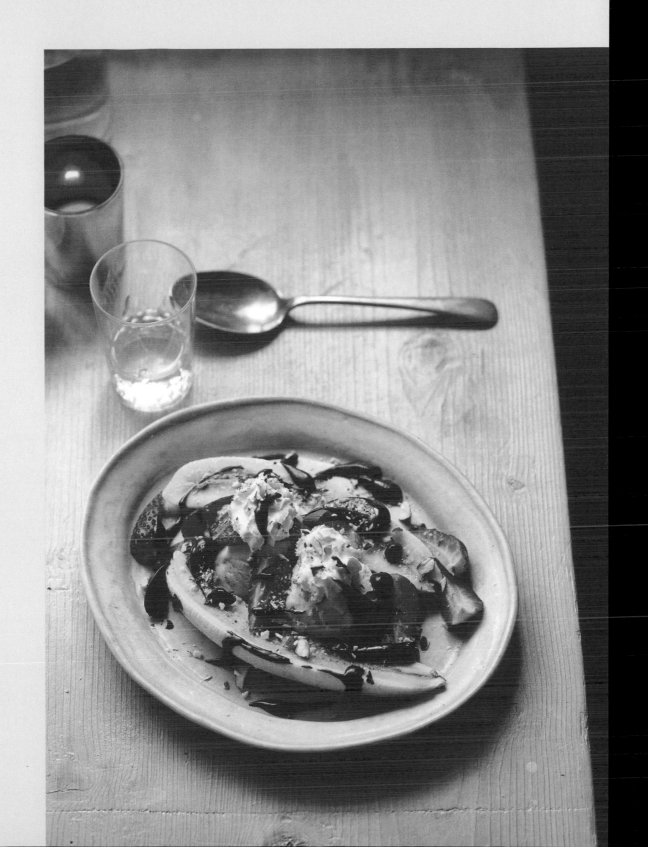

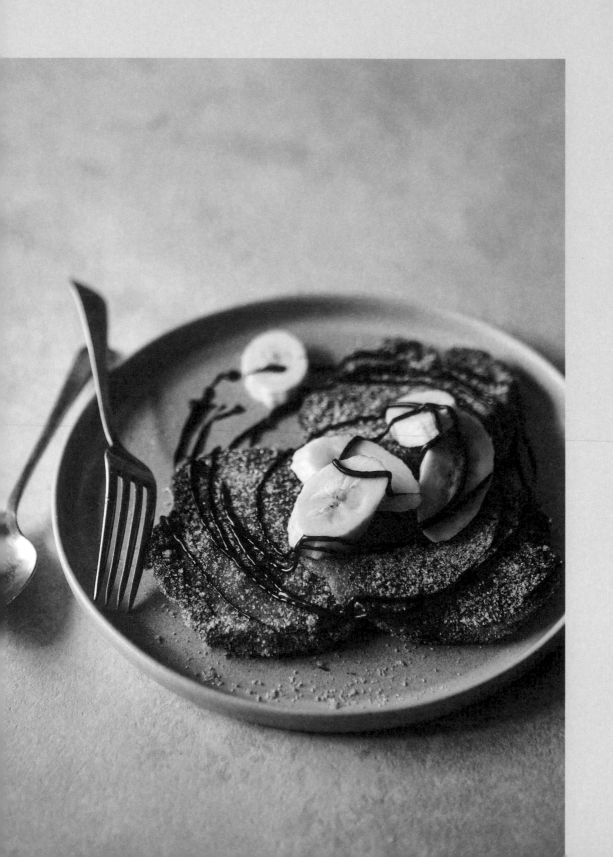

Churros Banana Fritters

This is different take on classic churros, but without the faff of the piping nozzle or deep-fat fryer. It is super simple, like making a pancake batter but with less liquid so it ends up as more of a fritter, which is crispy and crunchy. The cinnamon sugar is the perfect finishing touch and smells amazing when these are being cooked.

To make the batter, peel 3 of the bananas and mash with a fork in a large bowl until smooth. Sift in the flour, then crack in the egg and give everything a good mix to combine. You are looking for a thick batter that drops from the spoon, so check the consistency and stir though a splash of milk if the mixture is too thick.

Heat the oil in a large frying pan over a medium heat, then add 3 generous spoonfuls of the mixture set apart from each other to form 3 8-cm/3¼-inch fritters. Cook for around 2 minutes until the undersides are golden, then flip the fritters and cook for another 2 minutes until the fritters are golden all over. Remove from the pan to a sheet of kitchen paper to soak up any excess oil, then repeat the process to make another 3 fritters.

Combine the sugar and cinnamon in a shallow bowl, then, while the fritters are still hot from the pan, press them into the sugar mixture to coat.

Put the chocolate in heatproof bowl set over a pan of barely simmering water to melt, or put a microwavable bowl and melt in the microwave in short bursts. Peel and slice the remaining banana.

Divide the fritters between four serving plates (I like to give 2 to adults and 1 to children, but you could give everyone 1½ each if you're feeling generous!). Divide the sliced banana between the plates and frizzle over the melted chocolate. Serve while the fritters are still warm.

Prep: 5 minutes
Cook: 5 minutes
Serves 4

4 ripe bananas
100 g/3½ oz self-raising flour
1 large egg
splash of milk (optional)
100 ml/3½ fl oz sunflower or
    vegetable oil
1 tsp ground cinnamon
100 g/3½ oz caster sugar
50 g/2 oz dark chocolate, broken
    into squares

For first-stage weaning:
Omit the sugar and chocolate drizzle, then slice the fritters into batons and serve as a finger food with some chopped banana alongside

For older children:
Older children can enjoy these as they are for an occasional treat.

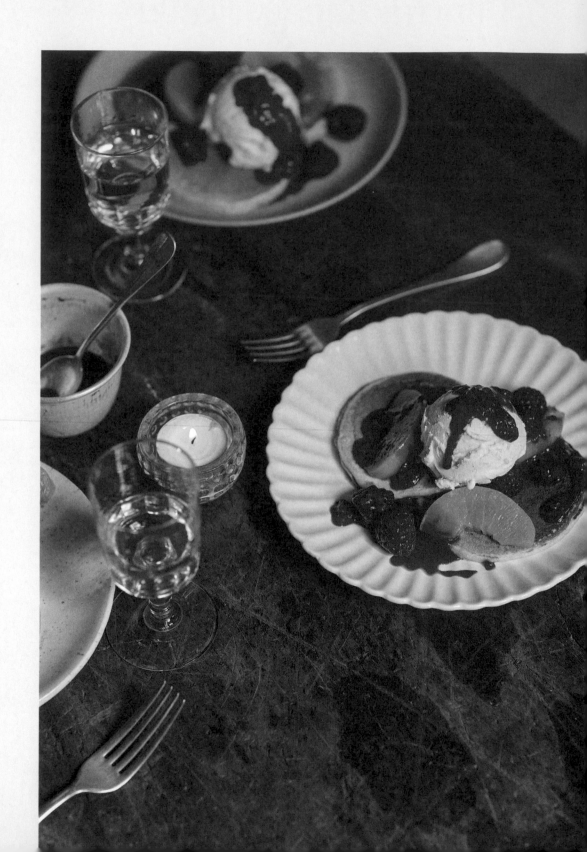

Peach Melba Pancakes

I have put my favourite breakfast pancakes in the Breakfasts section, but I couldn't also not include a dessert pancake option. These are peach melba-inspired and pack a punch that kids and adults alike will love. If anyone wants to know what to serve the mums in the house on Mother's Day, these are a fab choice (hint hint, Marvin!)

Place a sieve or colander over a bowl and strain the can of peaches through it, reserving the syrup. Put 200 g/7 oz of the drained peaches in a blender jug, setting aside the remainder to use when serving the pancakes. Add the egg, flour, milk, and desiccated coconut to the jug and blend the mixture to a smooth batter.

Put a large frying pan over a medium heat and melt the coconut oil. Once the oil is hot, add 3 generous ladlefuls of the mixture set apart from each other to form 3 6 cm/2½ inch pancakes. Cook for around 2–3 minutes until the undersides are golden, then flip the pancakes and cook the top sides for another 2 minutes until golden. Remove from the pan and keep warm while you repeat the process until all of the batter is used up (you should have enough batter to make 8 pancakes).

Put 50 g/1¾ oz of the raspberries in a microwavable bowl and microwave on high for 30 seconds until the raspberries break down and start to look pulpy. Stir through a couple of tablespoons of the reserved peach syrup, to taste.

Divide the pancakes between serving plates and top each with a dollop of yoghurt or a scoop of ice cream, a drizzle of raspberry sauce, a scattering of fresh raspberries, the reserved canned peaches and a little more of the reserved peach syrup.

Prep: 5 minutes
Cook: 10 minutes
Serves 4

1 x 400 g/14 oz can peaches in syrup
1 large egg
125 g/4½ oz self-raising flour
50 ml/2 fl oz semi-skimmed milk
2 tbsp desiccated coconut
2 tbsp coconut oil
250 g/9 oz raspberries
200 g/7 oz natural yoghurt or
   4 scoops vanilla ice cream

For first-stage weaning:
Substitute the canned peaches in syrup for peaches in juice, which have a lower sugar content. Blitz some of the drained peaches with a little yoghurt to make a purée.

For older children:
Substitute the canned peaches in syrup for peaches in juice, which have a lower sugar content. Older children will enjoy this as it is or, for toddlers, slice the pancakes into batons and serve with yoghurt alongside for dipping into.

Rice Pudding
with Blueberries

Prep: 5 minutes
Cook: 30-35 minutes
Serves 4

200 g/7 oz pudding rice
50 g/1¾ oz golden caster sugar
600 ml/1 pint whole milk
150 g/5½ oz fresh or frozen
  blueberries
juice of 1 orange

For first-stage weaning:
For babies and children under
12 months, omit the sugar, but
otherwise serve this as it is.

For older children:
Older children can enjoy a small
portion of this for dessert.

Some puddings never go out of style and this is one
of them. This creamy and indulgent recipe is fool-proof
and gets rave reviews from Marvin and the kids alike.

Rinse the rice under cold running water until the water runs
clear. Bring a pan of water to the boil over a medium heat,
then tip in the rice and cook for 2-3 minutes to start the
cooking process. Drain the rice through a colander, then return
the empty pan to the heat and add the sugar, 400 ml/
14 fl oz of the milk and the part-cooked rice. Bring the mixture
to a simmer, then reduce the heat to low and cook, stirring
occasionally, for 20-25 minutes.

Add another 150 ml/5 fl oz of the milk to the rice pudding
mixture and stir to combine, then leave to cook for another
10 minutes until the mixture is creamy and the rice is tender.

Meanwhile, put the fresh or frozen blueberries and orange
juice in a small pan and place over a high heat. Bring to the
boil, then reduce the heat to a simmer and leave to cook for
2-3 minutes, stirring occasionally until the fruit has broken
down to form a hot blueberry and orange cômpote.

Stir the remaining 50 ml/2 fl oz of milk through the rice
pudding, to loosen, then spoon into serving bowls. Top each
bowl with a generous swirl of the blueberry compote and
serve while the pudding is still hot.

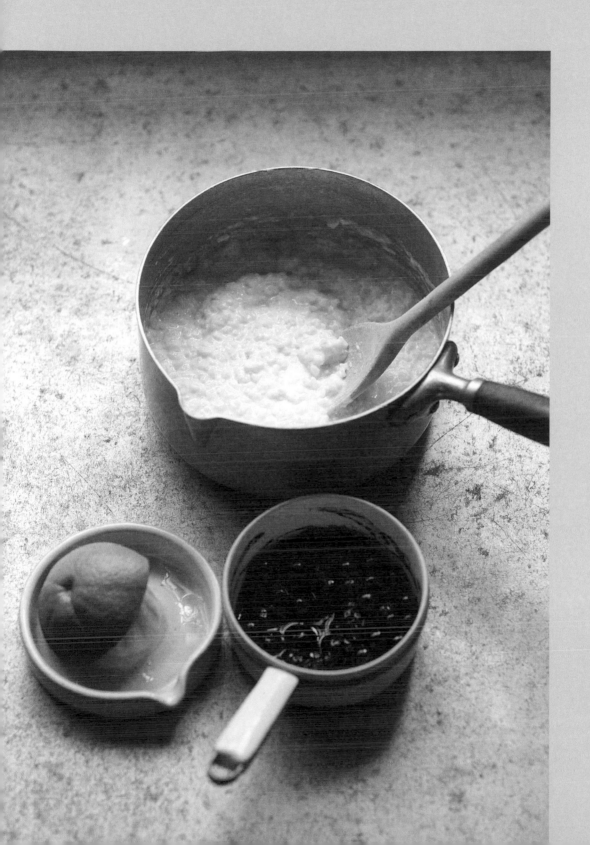

My go-to birthday cake!

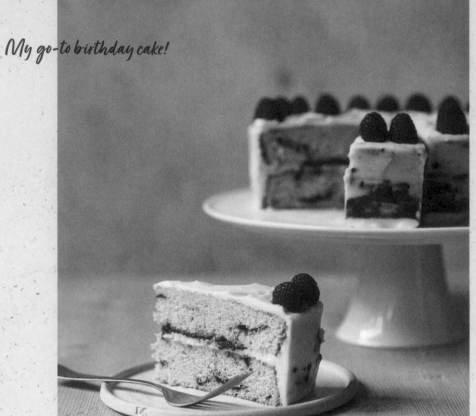

Here I have compiled a range of delicious occasion meals all in one place. We love hosting our friends and family and always try to create the best party menus. Whether you are looking for a showstopping dessert for a special occasion (see my Salted Caramel Pavlova on page 196) or you simply want something savoury to serve with drinks, here are my favourite options for those memorable days.

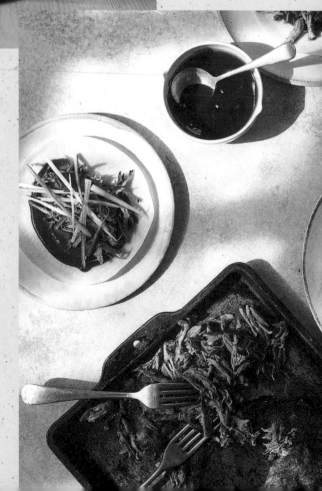

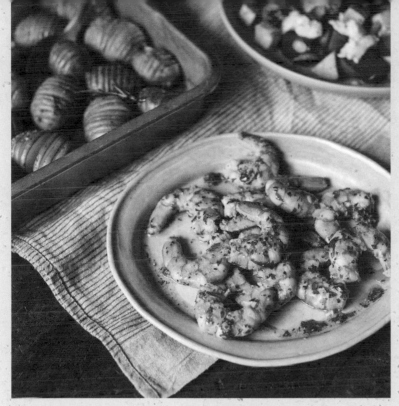

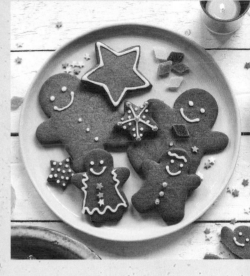

Occasions

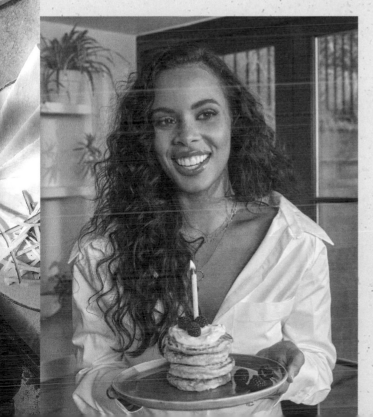

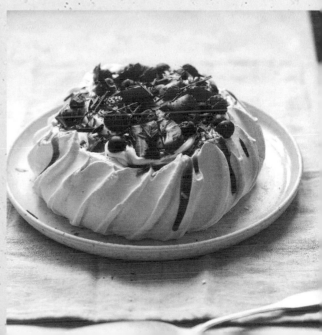

These prawns are one of my favourite things to eat, particularly during the summer months. I will serve them to friends at a barbecue, as a refreshing starter at a dinner party or, as here, paired with potatoes and salad as a meal in their own right. They are a great crowd-pleaser, but sometimes I will even make them for lunch when I am on my own and fancy a treat!

For first-stage weaning:
Cooked thoroughly, prawns can be introduced from 6 months, along with other potential allergens. Adapt the meal by boiling, rather than roasting, the potatoes, then mashing up with some unseasoned, cooked prawns and some chopped avocado.

For older children:
Older children can enjoy this as it is, just omit the salt and pepper when preparing the food and pass it around to the adults only when serving.

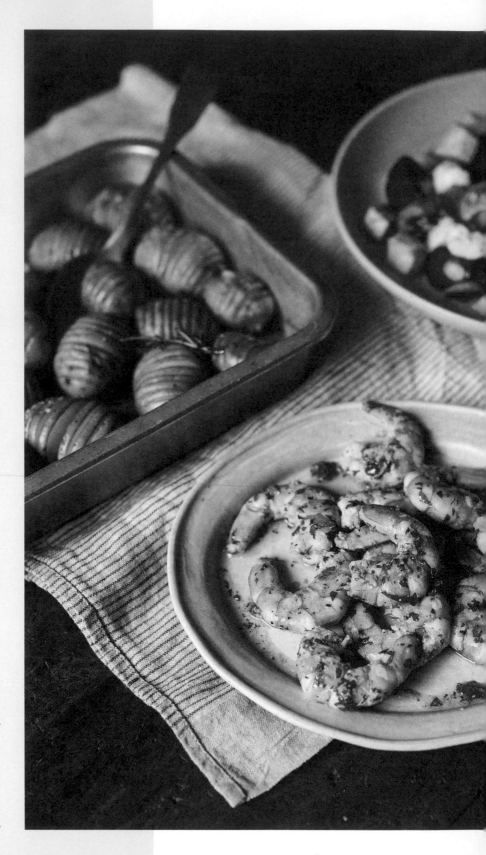

Garlic Prawns with Hasselback Potatoes & Hearty Salad

Preheat the oven to 180°C/350°F/gas mark 4.

Lay 2 chopsticks parallel to each other on a chopping board. One at a time, place the potatoes between the chopsticks and slice down through them at 5 mm/¼ inch intervals along their lengths, using the chopsticks as a barrier to prevent you from slicing all of the way through. Repeat until all of the potatoes are sliced.

Arrange the potatoes cut-side up in a roasting tin and drizzle with 3 tablespoons of the olive oil and a generous grinding of salt and pepper. Use the rosemary sprigs to brush the oil over the potatoes, ensuring they are well coated, then lay them over the top. Transfer to the oven for 40–50 minutes until crisp and golden.

Meanwhile, arrange the tomatoes on a large serving platter, ensuring that larger tomatoes are quartered and smaller ones are cut into halves. Finely chop most of the basil leaves, reserving a few whole leaves to use as a garnish, then scatter the chopped basil over the tomatoes. Lay the avocado slices over the top of the tomatoes, then tear over the mozzarella. Season the salad with salt and pepper, then drizzle with the 2 tablespoons of the oil and garnish with the reserved basil leaves. Set aside while you prepare the prawns.

Heat the remaining tablespoon of oil in a frying pan over a medium heat. Add the garlic and cook, stirring, for 30 seconds to soften, being careful not to burn. Add the prawns, chopped parsley and lemon juice and cook, stirring, for 5 minutes until the prawns are pink and cooked through. Season with salt, pepper and a pinch of chilli flakes, if using, then transfer the prawns to a serving plate. Put the prawns, salad and potatoes in the centre of the table and let everyone dig in and serve themselves.

Prep: 15 minutes
Cook: 40 minutes
Serves 6-8

1.5 kg/3 lb new potatoes
6 tbsp extra-virgin olive oil
6 sprigs fresh rosemary
1 kg/2 lb 4 oz mixed tomatoes,
   cut into halves or quarters
small bunch basil, leaves picked
2 ripe avocados, peeled, stoned and
   sliced
225 g/9 oz mozzarella
3 garlic cloves, crushed
600 g/1 lb 5 oz raw peeled king
   prawns
small bunch flat leaf parsley,
   leaves chopped
juice of 1 lemon
pinch of chilli flakes (optional)
sea salt and freshly ground
   black pepper

Crispy Hoisin Duck & Pancakes

Prep: 2 minutes
Cook: 1 hour 30 minutes
Serves 4 (or 8 as a starter)

4 Gressingham duck legs (approx. 225 g/8 oz each)
4 tbsp Chinese five spice
4 star anise
sea salt and freshly ground black pepper
½ cucumber, finely sliced into batons
1 bunch spring onions, shredded
1 x 200g/7 oz jar hoisin sauce (check label for allergens)
juice of 1 lime
20 store-bought Chinese pancakes
sea salt

For first-stage weaning:
If you have very young children at the table, chop some of the cucumber into large batons and let them chew and nibble on that while you enjoy the duck. The meat and sauce are highly seasoned, so are not suitable for young children.

For older children:
A small portion of this should be fine for older children, just keep an eye that they are only helping themselves to a tiny bit of the sauce as it can be very salty.

This crispy duck and pancake recipe uses duck legs that are widely available in the supermarkets and are very easy to cook. I use a shop-bought hoisin sauce for ease, making this impressive dish actually super simple! This is perfect for dinner parties, Chinese New Year celebrations, or a Saturday night do-it-yourself takeaway alternative.

Preheat the oven to 150°C/300°F/gas mark 2.

Put the duck legs in a large bowl and sprinkle over the Chinese five spice and generous grinding of salt, turning legs in the seasoning to ensure they are well coated. Transfer the duck to a roasting tin, ideally on a trivet to keep the legs elevated. (The legs will release a lot of fat when cooking, so keeping them raised ensures that they crisp up.) Add the star anise to the tin, then transfer to the oven and cook for 1 hour, basting the duck with its fat halfway through.

After 1 hour, increase the oven temperature to 200°C/400°F/gas mark 6 and cook for another 30–35 minutes until the skin is crisp and golden.

Meanwhile, put the sliced cucumber and spring onions in small bowls. Pour the hoisin into a bowl, add the lime juice and stir to combine. Heat the pancakes according to the packet instructions and cover with a cloth to keep warm. Place all of the elements in the middle of the table.

Transfer the duck to a serving plate, then use 2 forks to shred the meat. Put the meat in the middle of the table, then allow everyone to dig in and assemble their own pancakes.

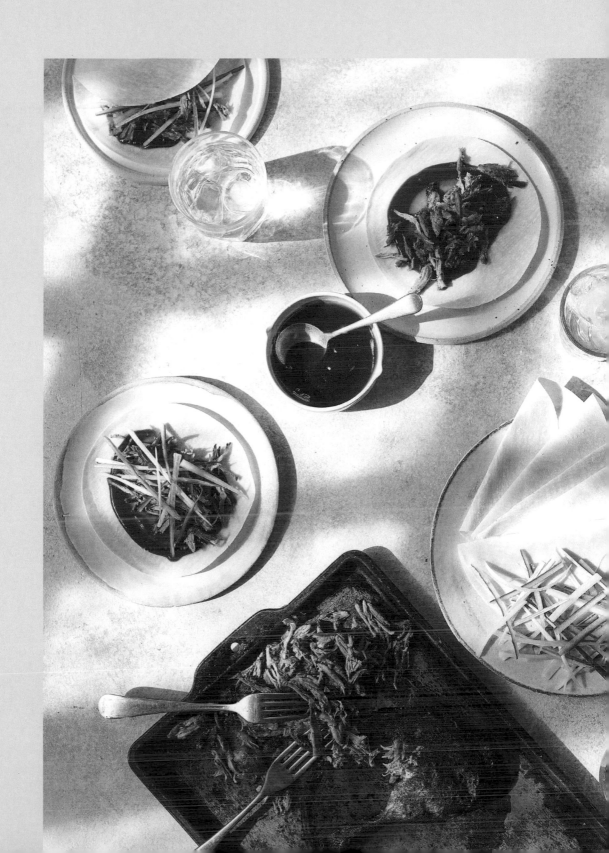

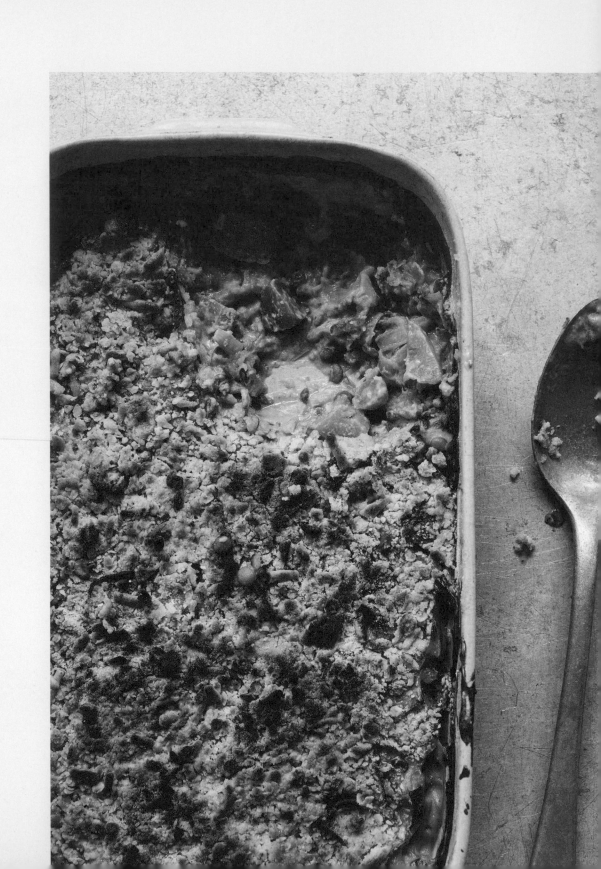

Veggie Crumble

This is a really filling and warming dish and a great way to get more veggies into the kids. Carrots and butternut squash are packed with good stuff, but you can switch up the filling if you have different seasonal veg in the cupboard or fridge that needs to be used. As well as for special occasions, I will sometimes cook this dish for a midweek family meal.

Preheat the oven to 200°C/400°F/gas mark 6.

To make the crumble topping, sift the flour into a large bowl and add the butter. Using your fingers, rub the butter into the flour until the mixture resembles breadcrumbs, then add the grated cheese and porridge oats to the bowl and stir to combine. Set aside.

To make the filling, melt the butter in a pan over a medium heat, then add the flour and cook, stirring continuously, for 1–2 minutes, to make a thick paste. Add a little of the milk and stir into the flour mixture until thickened, then keep adding the milk in stages, stirring and thickening between each addition until you have a thick, glossy sauce. Add the grated cheese, season with salt and pepper and stir until the cheese has melted through, then add the onion, carrots, garlic, squash and leek, and cook, stirring occasionally, for 5 minutes. Stir the drained lentils and chopped parsley through the sauce, then pour the mixture into a large baking dish. Scatter the crumble over the top in an even layer to cover, then transfer to the oven and bake for 30–40 minutes until golden and bubbling. Serve hot, with steamed broccoli on the side.

Prep: 10 minutes
Cook: 50 minutes
Serves 4

35 g/1¼ oz unsalted butter
2 tbsp plain flour
500 ml/18 fl oz whole milk
35 g/1¼ oz Cheddar cheese
1 red onion, halved and finely sliced
1 garlic clove, crushed
2 carrots, peeled and chopped
300 g/10½ oz butternut squash, peeled and cut into 2 cm/¾ in chunks
1 leek, cut into 2 cm/¾ in slices
1 x 400g can cooked lentils, drained
small bunch flat leaf parsley, leaves roughly chopped
sea salt and freshly ground black pepper
steamed broccoli, to serve

For the crumble topping:
100 g/3½ oz plain flour
500 g/1 lb 2 oz fridge-cold unsalted butter, cubed
25 g/1 oz Cheddar cheese
25 g/1 oz porridge oats

For first-stage weaning:
Cook the veg in the white sauce until tender, omitting seasoning from the sauce, then blend to a purée. Serve with some steamed broccoli alongside for chewing and holding.

For older children:
Older children will enjoy the crumble as it is.

Fun Festive Party Ideas

When you have lots of people round for an informal party you want something fun and simple that isn't going to eat up your time and pull you away from your guests. These recipes are sure to be crowd pleasers for party goers of any age and almost all of the work can be done in advance, keeping you out of the kitchen!

Honey & Mustard Chipolatas

Prep: 5 minutes
Cook: 15 minutes

24 chipolata sausages
4 tbsp clear honey
4 tsp Dijon mustard
sea salt

For first-stage weaning:
Honey is unsuitable for children below 12 months, so skip the sauce and just serve the grilled sausages cut up into chunks.

For older children:
Older children will enjoy these as they are.

Do you ever struggle with ideas on what to serve with drinks? Are you looking for an easy party food option? These honey and mustard sausages have a lovely sticky and sweet taste – one nibble at a time or ten, these will always disappear very quickly. They're also a great for the kids' tea.

Preheat the grill to high and line a large roasting tin with foil.

Put the chipolatas in the prepared roasting tin, then place under the grill for 5 minutes.

Meanwhile, combine the honey, mustard and a pinch of salt in a bowl. After 5 minutes, remove the sausages from under the grill and pour over the sauce, stirring to ensure that the sausages are well coated.

Return the roasting tin to under the grill and cook for another 10 minutes, turning halfway through until the sausages are sticky, golden and cooked through. Transfer the chipolatas to a serving dish and serve with cocktail sticks on the side, so that people can easily grab them without getting sticky fingers!

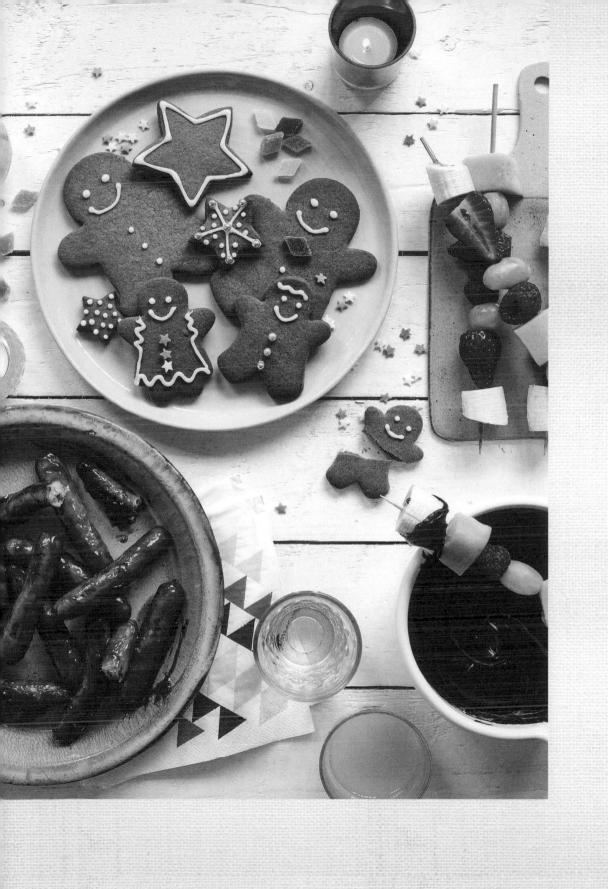

Gingerbread Biscuits

This is the only gingerbread recipe that you will ever need! This recipe is an easy one to bake with the kids and is ideal for play-date fun or for kids' parties. My kids love adding the icing and decorations. These also keep for ages and can be kept in airtight containers. We love baking this recipe at Christmas and taking our neighbours some of the biscuits as a gift.

Prep: 10 minutes
Cook: 10 minutes
Makes 50 (depending on size)

180 g/6 oz unsalted butter, cubed
150 g/6 oz dark muscovado sugar
80 g/3 oz golden syrup
450 g/1 lb plain flour
½ tbsp bicarbonate of soda
1 tbsp ground ginger
1 tbsp ground cinnamon

For the icing and decoration:
300 g/10½ oz icing sugar
4 tbsp water
sprinkles, edible glitter and jelly
   sweets, to decorate

For first-stage weaning:
The sugar in these makes them unsuitable for very young children.

For older children:
Older children will love these, not least because they can get involved with choosing the shapes and decorating the biscuits.

Preheat the oven to 180°C/350°F/gas mark 4 and line several large baking sheets with greaseproof paper.

Heat the butter, sugar and golden syrup in a pan over a medium heat until the butter has melted and the sugar has dissolved.

Sift the flour, bicarbonate of soda, ginger and cinnamon into a large bowl and make a well in the centre. Pour the butter and syrup mixture into the well, then use a wooden spoon to stir the mixture until it comes together to a dough. Set aside for a couple of minutes until cool enough to handle, then turn out onto a lightly floured surface and bring the mixture together with your hands, being careful not to over-handle as this can result in a tough dough. Press the dough down into a flat disc, cover with plastic wrap and transfer it to the fridge to rest for 20 minutes.

Once rested, roll the dough out on a lightly floured surface to a thickness of 3 mm/⅛ inch (about the thickness of a £1 coin). Use cutters of your choice to stamp out biscuits, then transfer to the prepared baking sheets, leaving room between the biscuits to allow them to spread slightly during cooking. Re-roll the scraps to use up any remaining dough.

Transfer the biscuits to the oven and leave to bake for 10 minutes until light golden brown. Leave the biscuits on the trays for 10 minutes to firm up, then transfer to a wire rack to cool.

While the biscuits are cooling, make the icing. Sift the icing sugar into a large bowl, gradually add the water and whisk or stir to combine to a thick icing; if the icing is too thin it will just run off the biscuits. Put the icing into piping bags and snip off the ends, then decorate the biscuits as you would like (or ask your kids to come and help!). Add sprinkles, edible glitter and jelly sweets to finish. Set aside for a few minutes to allow the icing to set, then the biscuits are ready to enjoy! These will keep for several weeks in an airtight container.

Chocolate Fondue & Fruit Skewers

This is such a fun dessert option and is popular with both the kids and adults. Amazingly, it will even count towards your five-a-day! It is also a great way of encouraging the kids to try new fruits or encourage them to try ones that they are unsure about.

Put the chocolate, butter, cream and milk in a pan over a low heat and cook, stirring continuously until the chocolate and butter have melted and everything has come together to a smooth, silky sauce. Transfer to a deep serving dish, or leave in the pan and place in the middle of the table.

Thread the fruit onto wooden skewers, or put in a large bowl with the skewers alongside so that your guests can create their own. Serve the fondue, allowing guests to dip and drizzle their fruit in the chocolate sauce.

Prep: 15 minutes
Cook: 5 minutes
Serves 20

300 g/10½ oz 80% dark chocolate, broken into squares
80 g/3 oz unsalted butter, cubed
200 ml/7 fl oz double cream
150 ml/5 fl oz whole milk

For the fruit skewers:
400 g/14 oz strawberries, hulled and halved
125 g/4½ oz raspberries
1 ripe mango, halved, peeled and chopped into bite-sized pieces
2 ripe bananas, peeled and cut into 2 cm/¾ in slices
250 g/9 oz green grapes (halved if serving to young children)

For first-stage weaning:
Simply serve some of the fruit mashed down into a little yoghurt or as finger foods for older babies.

For older children:
This can be served as is, simply cut the fruit small enough so that it doesn't pose any choking hazards. Supervise children when eating as the skewers are sharp.

This show-stopping fruity cake always goes down a treat and it is ideal for summer days. This is lovely and succulent, and the ripples of raspberry in the sponge look really impressive when cut. This is my go-to when I am baking for baby showers, summer afternoon teas, sports days or birthdays.

For first-stage weaning: This is too sweet for very young children. Simply serve them some raspberries for a sweet treat.

For older children: A small slice of this is fine for older children to enjoy as an occasional treat or at a celebration.

Raspberry Ripple Cake

Preheat the oven to 180°C/350°F/gas mark 4 and grease a deep 25 cm/10 inch cake tin with butter and line with greaseproof paper.

To make the raspberry sauce, put 200 g/7 oz of the raspberries and 50 g/1¾ oz of golden caster sugar in a pan over a medium heat. Bring the mixture to the boil, then reduce to a simmer and cook, stirring occasionally, for 10 minutes until jammy. Set a coarse metal sieve over a bowl and press the raspberry sauce through it to remove any pips. Set aside.

To make the cake, beat the butter and sugar together with an electric whisk or in the bowl of a stand mixer until pale and fluffy. Crack in the eggs one at a time, beating and incorporating into the butter mixture between each addition. Add the milk and beat again to combine. Sift the flour and baking powder into the mixture, then add the ground almonds and mix again until everything is well combined.

Tip half of the cake batter into the prepared cake tin and level out with a spatula. Drizzle half of the raspberry sauce over, then use the back of a spoon to gently swirl it through the batter (don't be too heavy handed here, you are looking for swirls of raspberry, rather than turning the whole cake pink!). Pour the remaining cake batter over the top, then level out and swirl through the remaining raspberry sauce in the same way. Transfer to the oven and leave to bake for 50–60 minutes until the cake is golden, well risen and an inserted skewer comes out clean. Leave to cool in the tin for 10 minutes, then turn out onto a wire rack and leave to cool to room temperature.

While the cake is cooling, make the icing by sifting the icing sugar into a bowl or the bowl of a stand mixer and adding the butter. Beat with an electric whisk until the mixture has come together to form a paste, then add the cream cheese and beat on a low speed until smooth and creamy.

Once the cake has completely cooled, use a serrated knife to slice it in half. Put one of the halves, cut-side up, on a serving plate or cake board and spread with 2 tablespoons of raspberry jam. Spoon a third of the icing over and use a spatula to spread to the edges of the cake. Place the other half of the cake on the top, cut-side down. Gently swirl the remaining icing with 2 tablespoons of raspberry jam, then use this to coat the top and sides of the cake in a thin layer. Decorate the top of the cake with fresh raspberries, then slice and serve.

Prep: 20 minutes
Cook: 1 hour
Serves 16

250 g/9 oz room-temperature unsalted butter, cubed
450 g/1 lb golden caster sugar
6 large eggs
150 ml/5 fl oz whole milk
350 g/12 oz plain flour
2 tsp baking powder
85 g/3 oz ground almonds

For the raspberry sauce:
200 g/7 oz fresh raspberries
50 g/1¾ oz golden caster sugar

For the icing and decoration:
350 g/12 oz icing sugar
150 g/5½ room-temperature unsalted butter, cubed
250 g/9 oz full-fat cream cheese
3 heaped tbsp raspberry jam
150 g/5½ oz fresh raspberries

Salted Caramel Pavlova

Prep: 25 minutes
Cook: 1 hour
Serves 12

6 large eggs
300 g/10½ oz golden caster sugar
200 ml/7 fl oz double cream
400 g/14 oz Greek yoghurt
1 tsp vanilla paste
40 g/1½ oz 70% dark chocolate
400 g/14 oz strawberries, raspberries
  and blueberries

For the salted caramel sauce:
100 g/3½ oz golden caster sugar
50 g/1¾ oz unsalted butter, cubed
5 tbsp double cream
good pinch of sea salt flakes

For first-stage weaning:
This is too sweet for little tummies, so simply serve very young children some of the fruit mashed up with a little Greek yoghurt.

For older children:
As an occasional treat, older children can enjoy a slice of the pavlova without the caramel sauce. If they really want to try the caramel, make it without using salt and serve sparingly.

Preheat the oven to 150°C/300°F/gas mark 2 and line a large baking sheet with greaseproof paper.

Crack the eggs and separate the whites from the yolks. Using a stand mixer or electric whisk, whisk the egg whites at high speed until they form stiff peaks. With the whisk still running, start adding the sugar a spoonful at a time, leaving a few seconds between each addition to allow the sugar to incorporate. Once all of the sugar has been added, keep whisking on full speed for another 8 minutes until the meringue is stiff and glossy, and no grains of sugar can be felt when you rub the meringue between your fingers.

Tip the meringue onto your prepared baking sheet and form into a 23 cm/9 inch circle. For an extra flourish, swirl the meringue with the back of a spatula for a decorative effect, if you like. Transfer to the oven and bake for 1½ hours until lightly golden, then turn off the oven and leave the pavlova inside to cool and firm up for at least 2 hours. I like to cook the pavlova the night before I want to serve it and leave it in the oven to cool down slowly overnight.

About an hour before you want to serve your meringue, make the salted caramel sauce. Put the sugar in a heavy-based pan over a medium heat and leave to melt, swirling the pan from time to time, but not touching with a spoon. Once the sugar has all melted and is nice and golden, add the butter and whisk to combine. (Be careful here as the hot sugar will bubble up when you add the butter.) Once the butter has melted, add the cream and whisk again to combine. Leave to cook for another 2–3 minutes, then remove the pan from the heat and set aside to cool for 10 minutes. After 10 minutes, add a generous pinch of sea salt to the caramel and stir to combine. Set aside until you are ready to serve the pavlova.

Whisk the double cream with an electric whisk or in a stand mixer until it forms soft peaks, then fold in the yoghurt and vanilla paste. Put the pavlova on a serving plate, then spoon the cream and yoghurt mixture over the top. Chop the fruit and spoon that over also, then drizzle over the caramel sauce. Drag the blade of a sharp knife over the chocolate to create shavings, then sprinkle over the pavlova. Slice and serve.

If you are looking for an impressive dessert to dish up to friends and family, this is it! If you want to, you can make the meringue in advance. Sometimes pavlovas can be tricky, but this one is easy. Simply put this one on the table after dinner and let everyone dig in.

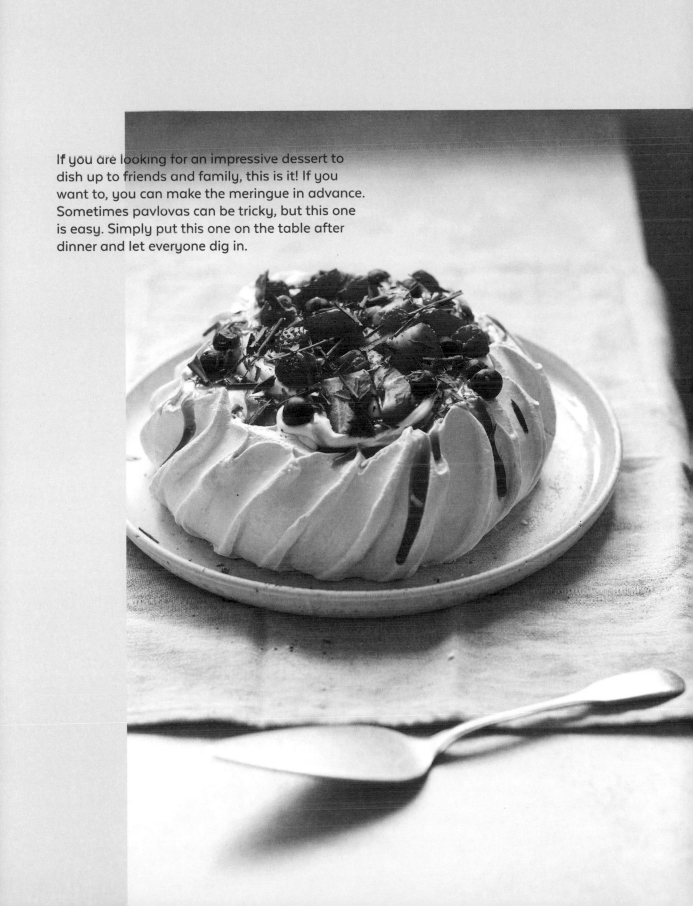

Creating Food Traditions

I really enjoy sitting down and getting together over food with my family, and many of our food traditions have been passed down through the generations. These traditions teach children that food isn't something to be rushed or eaten on the go, but can be a time to come together as a family and spend some real quality time.

* **Always have a special meal on Saturday or Sunday**: We have always cooked a roast or special meal on a Sunday. The day starts with chopping and peeling in the morning and goes from there, and it feels like a real ritual. I always cook meat with all the trimmings (see page 75) but there are plenty of other great options in this book for having a special meal together.

* **Pass favourite recipes down to the children**: When I first starting dating Marvin, his dad would cook us his special soup (see Pops' Saturday Soup on page 75) and we would go round on a Saturday and eat it together. It felt like quite a big deal when he trusted me with the recipe as I started making it at my house and his family would come to us. At some point we will teach it to Alaia, Valle and Blake, and they will continue the lovely tradition.

* **Birthday food**: From birthday cakes to meals out, I think it is important to have special food traditions on a birthday. Birthdays in our house always start with pancakes for breakfast!

* **Turn off the TV and take the phones away from the table when eating**: We always make a real point of not having our phones or any screens at the table. When we are out for the dinner with our family and friends, the phones go into the middle of the table and the first person to touch their phone has to pay the tip! When we are with our family, meals have always been the occasion when everyone catches up and chats about work and school.

* **Celebrate food from other cultures**: Broadening your food horizons and celebrating food from around the world is a great way of exploring different cultures. My particular favourites are Asian and Italian food. I think it's really important to introduce the kids to different foods early, so they get used to many different flavours.

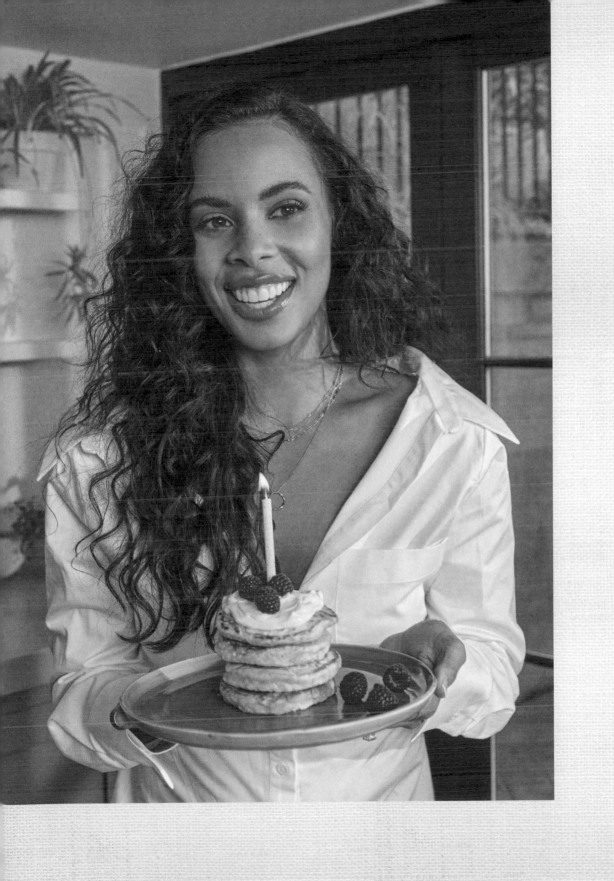

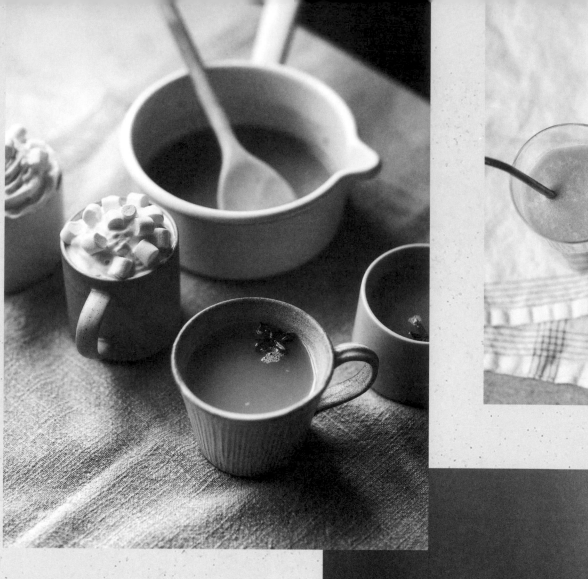

*No day is complete without the right drink in hand. Whether you are wanting a warming drink like a Hot Chocolate Orange (see page 205), something more fruity and summery like a Sunshine Smoothie (see page 209) or one of my special Fruity Mocktails (see page 210), this chapter has got you covered. A lot of these drinks are treats that I save for special nights, like dinner parties with friends or celebration meals, but there are plenty of healthy options, too. I hope you enjoy these as much as we do.

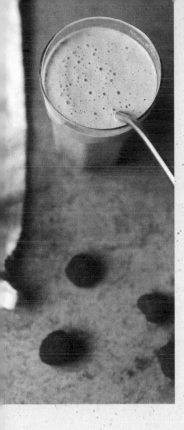

Drinks

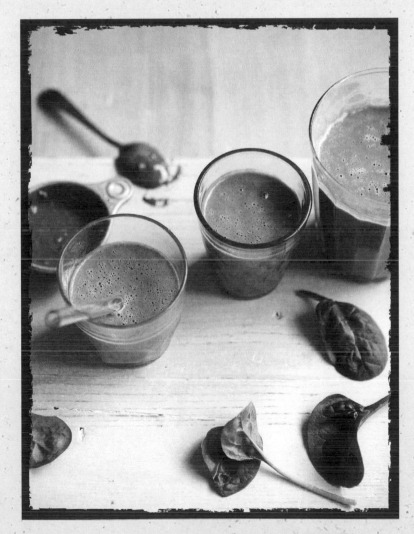

Looks healthy – tastes like white chocolate!

Easy Pink Lemonade

Prep: 5 minutes, plus cooling
Cook: 5 minutes
Serves 6-8

10 lemons
150 g/5 oz raspberries
125 g/4½ oz caster sugar
1 litre/1¾ pints boiling water

Note:
Because of the sugar content, this is unsuitable for children under 5 years old.

Tart and tasty, this recipe makes me think of hot summer days in the garden when the sun is blazing and the kids are splashing around in the paddling pool! Adding raspberries to traditional lemonade will turn it pink and give it an amazing, sweet flavour.

Using a vegetable peeler, remove the zest from 2 of the lemons and add to a large pan. Juice all the lemons and add the juice to the pan, then add the raspberries and caster sugar. Using a potato masher, mash everything together to break down the raspberries, then pour in the boiling water. Put the pan over a medium heat, bring to the boil then reduce the heat to a gentle simmer. Cook for 2–3 minutes, then turn off the heat and set aside for an hour or so until the lemonade is completely cool.

Once cooled, strain the lemonade through a fine sieve into a jug. Generously fill serving glasses with ice, then pour over the lemonade and serve immediately.

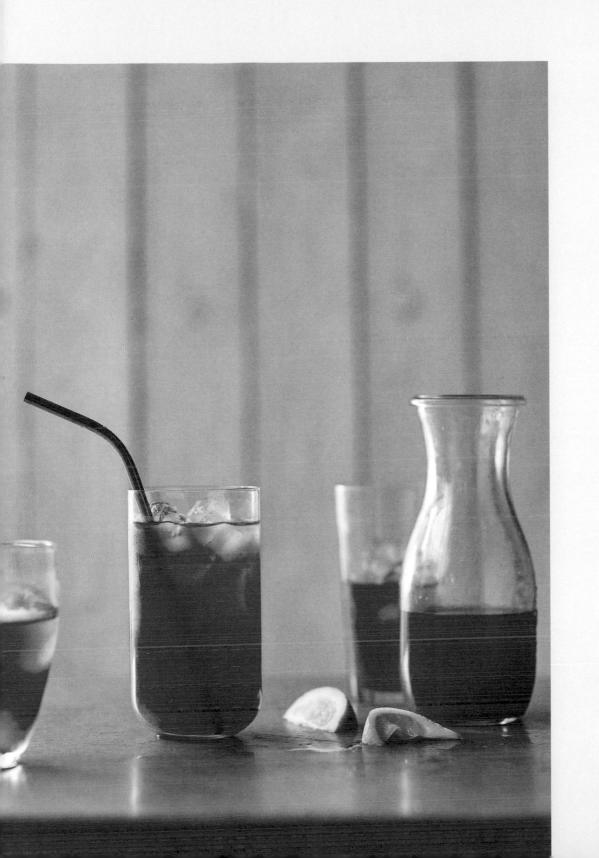

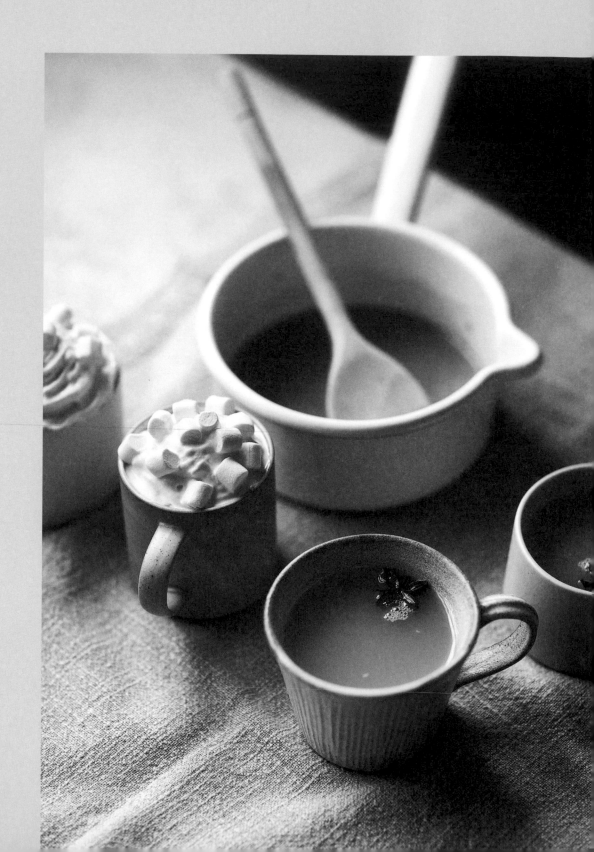

Hot Chocolate Orange

This is a real indulgent treat, especially if you go all out and add squirty cream and marshmallows. If you happen to have any classic chocolate orange around, add a few chunks to the pan to melt for an extra orangey hit.

Prep: 5 minutes
Serves 4

1 orange
4 tbsp hot chocolate powder
1 litre/1¾ pints whole milk
squirty cream
40 g/1½ oz mini marshmallows
10 g/¼ oz dark chocolate, grated

Zest the orange and juice half of it, then add the juice and zest to a pan. Add the hot chocolate powder and 4 tablespoons of the milk, then stir the mixture to a smooth paste. Pour in the remaining milk, then put the pan over a medium heat and cook, whisking continuously, for 5 minutes until steaming hot. If the milk begins to boil, reduce the heat to a gentle simmer.

Divide the hot chocolate between 4 mugs and top each with a few of the marshmallows, reserving some of the marshmallows for later. Top the mugs with a generous squirt of cream, then add the remaining marshmallows and finish with a few gratings of dark chocolate. Serve hot.

Note:
Because of the sugar content, this is unsuitable for children under 12 months old. For younger children, omit the marshmallows when serving.

Hot Spiced Apple Juice

This is a bit like a mulled apple juice, with a kick of ginger and optional booze! This is a great drink that the whole family can enjoy on cold winter nights.

Prep: 5 minutes
Serves 2

500 ml/18 fl oz apple juice
1 tsp grated fresh ginger
2 star anise
1 cinnamon stick
4 tbsp rum or whisky (optional)

Put the apple juice, ginger, star anise and cinnamon stick in a pan over a medium heat, bring to the boil, then reduce to a simmer, add the rum or whisky, if using, and leave to cook for 3 minutes to let the flavours develop. Strain the mixture into mugs, picking out the star anise and adding to the mugs also, then serve warm.

Angie's Fraud Shake

Prep: 2 minutes
Serves 2

200 g/7 oz fresh mango, cut
   into chunks
1 tbsp peanut butter
1 tsp clear honey
100 g/3½ oz spinach
200 ml/7 fl oz oat milk
200 ml/7 fl oz water

Note:
This contains honey, so is
unsuitable for children younger
than 12 months.

This is my friend Angie's recipe. It might sound strange, but put all these ingredients together and you get something that tastes bizarrely like white chocolate! The spinach does give this a green tinge, but once your kids taste it, you'll never look back!

Put all of the ingredients in a blender, then blend until smooth. Pour the shake into 2 tall, ice-filled glasses and enjoy!

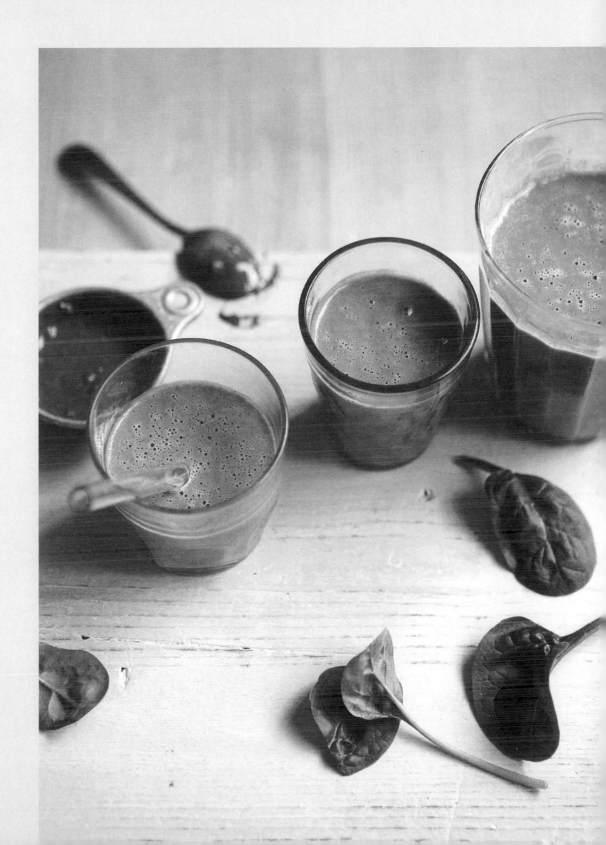

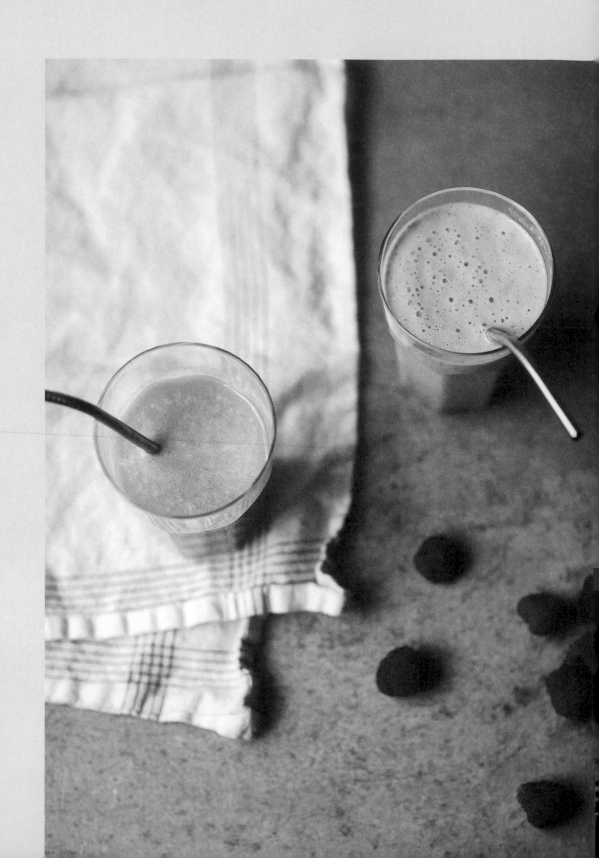

Red Berry Smoothie

Fruit-packed smoothies feel like a treat, but are a great way of getting some extra goodness into the kids. This one has strawberries, bananas and raspberries, with no added sugar – just a drizzle of honey. Use whatever berries are in season. This is lovely and filling, so makes a great addition to the breakfast table to keep appetites, big and small, satisfied until lunch.

Hull the strawberries and add to a blender along with the raspberries, banana and milk. Blend until smooth, then taste and add a little honey to sweeten, if needed. Blend the smoothie again, then pour into serving glasses and serve immediately.

Prep: 5 minutes
Serves 2

100 g/3½ oz fresh strawberries
100 g/3½ oz frozen raspberries
1 banana, peeled and sliced
250 ml/9 fl oz whole milk
clear honey, to sweeten (optional)

Note:
If sweetened with honey, this is unsuitable for children younger than 12 months.

Sunshine Smoothie

This fruity smoothie is packed with sunshine and makes the ultimate summer cooler. Flaxseeds are packed with omega 3s and fibre and also help thicken the smoothie. You can get packs of mixed frozen tropical fruits in the supermarket, but if you don't particularly like pineapple or mango, just switch them out for other fresh or frozen fruit of your choice.

Put all the ingredients in a blender and blend until smooth. Pour the smoothie into 2 tall, ice-filled glasses and serve immediately.

Prep: 2 minutes
Serves 2

350 ml/12 fl oz fresh orange juice
100 g/3½ oz frozen mango, pineapple and papaya
1 tsp ground flaxseed

Fruity Mocktails

Prep: 5 minutes
Serves 2

2 pomegranates
1 orange
150 ml/5 fl oz apple juice
30 g/1 oz fresh raspberries
200 ml/7 fl oz tonic water

Note:
Pomegranate seeds can present a choking hazard for very young children, so this is unsuitable for those younger than 12 months.

There is nothing my kids love more than pretending to be all grown up. Here are three mocktail combos, which all have really different flavours and make perfect kids' drinks when they want to join in with the grown-ups. Of course, if you fancy it, they could be upgraded with a little gin, vodka or whatever your favourite spirit might be to make a special treat for Mum or Dad! I am definitely partial to a splash of gin in the Cucumber Fizz.

POMEGRANATE PUNCH

Cut the pomegranates in half, scoop the seeds out of 1 of the halves and set aside for later. Juice the remaining 3 halves (you need around 4 tablespoons of juice) and add the juice to a blender. Halve the orange, cut one of the halves into slices and set aside for later. Juice the remaining orange half and add the juice to the blender, along with the apple juice and fresh raspberries. Blend the mixture until smooth, then divide the mixture between 2 tall, ice-filled glasses. Top the glasses up with tonic water and serve the drinks garnished with the orange slices and pomegranate seeds.

CUCUMBER FIZZ

Put the cucumber in a cocktail shaker or jug along with the elderflower cordial and mint leaves. Squeeze in the juice from the lime, then throw in the lime halves, too. Add a handful of crushed ice, then, using a cocktail muddler or rolling pin, give everything a good muddle to extract as much flavour as possible from all of the elements. Pour in the soda water and give the mixture a stir to combine, then strain into 2 tall, ice-filled glasses and serve immediately.

Prep: 5 minutes
Serves 2

100 g/3½ oz cucumber, roughly
  chopped
150 ml/5 fl oz elderflower cordial
4 sprigs mint, leaves picked
1 lime, halved
300 ml/10 fl oz soda water

BLACKBERRY GINGER FOREST

Hold back a couple of blackberries or blueberries for garnishing and put the rest in a blender with a splash of the apple juice. Blend to a paste, then add the remaining apple juice and ginger beer, and give the mix a stir to combine. Pour the mixture into tall, ice-filled glasses and garnish with the reserved blackberries or blueberries and a couple of slices of apple, if using. Serve immediately.

Prep: 5 minutes
Serves 2

45 g/1¾ oz fresh blackberries
  or blueberries
200 ml/7 fl oz apple juice
200 ml/7 fl oz ginger beer
½ apple, thinly sliced, to garnish
  (optional)

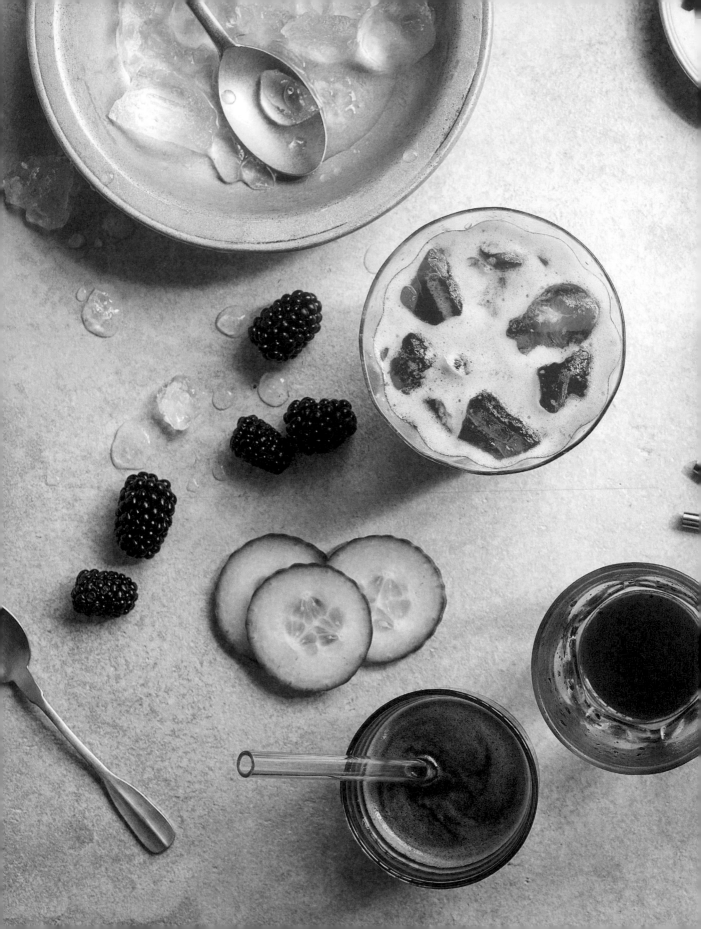

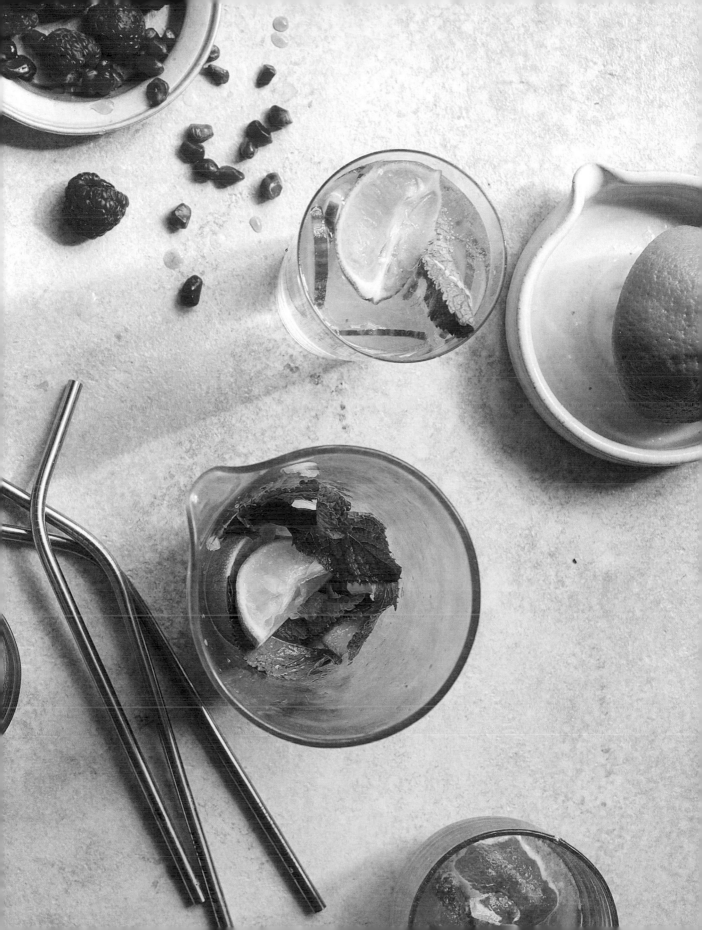

Banana & Strawberry Milkshake

Prep: 5 minutes
Serves 2

100 g/3½ oz frozen strawberries
1 banana, peeled and sliced
150 ml/5 fl oz oat milk
50 g/2 oz Greek yoghurt
clear honey, to sweeten (optional)

Note:
If sweetened with honey, this is
unsuitable for children younger
than 12 months.

An absolute treat for any time of the day, this milkshake will offer kids a blast of energy. Traditional milkshake recipes often include ice cream, but I've subbed in Greek yoghurt here, to make it a healthier option that is just as creamy and delicious. If you can't find frozen strawberries, just use fresh, hulled strawberries and add a handful of crushed ice to the blender when making the milkshake.

Put all the ingredients in a blender and blend until smooth. Taste the milkshake and add a little honey to sweeten, if needed, then blend the smoothie again, pour into glasses and serve immediately.

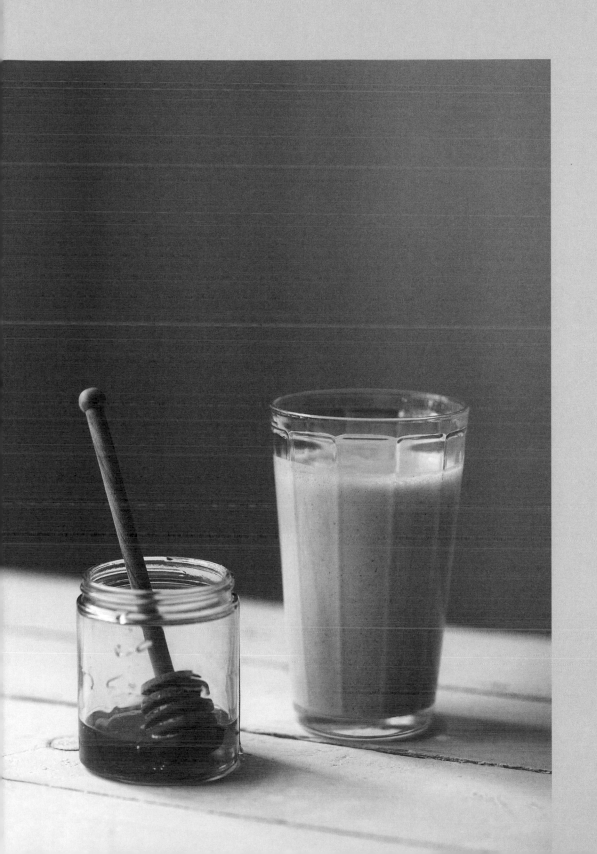

Handy Conversions

All of the recipes in this book list both metric and imperial measurements, but if you want to scale a recipe up or down or are cooking somewhere in the world where you're more used to using a different unit of measurement (cups, for example), you can use the information on these two pages to make any adjustments.

OVEN TEMPERATURES

Temperatures can vary between ovens, so it is worth checking that yours is running at the correct heat by testing with an oven thermometer. You may need to adjust the temperature if you know your oven runs particularly hot or cold. I cook in an electric fan oven, so if you use gas you may want to increase the oven temps slightly.

140°C	275°F	gas mark 1
150°C	300°F	gas mark 2
160°C	325°F	gas mark 3
180°C	350°F	gas mark 4
190°C	375°F	gas mark 5
200°C	400°F	gas mark 6
220°C	425°F	gas mark 7
230°C	450°F	gas mark 8
240°C	475°F	gas mark 9

WEIGHT CONVERSIONS

In the UK, we generally use metric (gram) measurements for dry ingredients, though some people prefer to use imperial (ounce) measurements. Most electronic cook's scales will happily do both, so use whichever you are happiest with.

25/30 g	1 oz
40 g	1½ oz
50 g	1¾ oz
55 g	2 oz
70 g	2½ oz
85 g	3 oz
100 g	3½ oz
115 g	4 oz
150 g	5½ oz
200 g	7 oz
225 g	8 oz
250 g	9 oz
300 g	10½ oz
350 g	12 oz
375 g	13 oz
400 g	14 oz
450 g	1 lb
500 g	1 lb 2 oz
600 g	1 lb 5 oz
750 g	1 lb 10 oz
900 g	2 lb
1 kg	2 lb 4 oz
2 kg	4 lb 8 oz

VOLUME CONVERSIONS

Wet ingredients, such as water, stock, oil and milk, are often measured in millilitres (ml) or fluid ounces (fl oz), though smaller amounts can be measured in teaspoons or tablespoons. Because these are worked out on volume as opposed to weight, it is very easy to work out an equivalent cup measurement.

5 ml	–	1 tsp
15 ml	½ fl oz	1 tbsp
30 ml	1 fl oz	2 tbsp
60 ml	2 fl oz	¼ cup
75 ml	2½ fl oz	⅓ cup
120 ml	4 fl oz	½ cup
150 ml	5 fl oz	⅔ cup
175 ml	6 fl oz	¾ cup
250 ml	8 fl oz	1 cup
350 ml	12 fl oz	1½ cups
500 ml	18 fl oz	2 cups
1 litre	1¾ pints	4 cups

CUP MEASURES FOR DRY INGREDIENTS

For dry ingredients, which are usually measured by weight, it is much harder to convert to a cup measurement as there is no universal rule (a cup of butter weighs much more than a cup of flour, for example). The list below gives an approximate cup equivalent to the some of the most commonly used ingredients that you may want to weigh in this way.

Flour	125 g	1 cup
Sugar (white)	200 g	1 cup
Sugar (brown)	200 g	1 cup
Sugar (icing)	130 g	1 cup
Butter	225 g	1 cup (2 sticks)
Breadcrumbs (dried)	125 g	1 cup
Nuts	125 g	1 cup
Seeds	160 g	1 cup
Dried fruit	150 g	1 cup
Pasta (dried penne)	90 g	1 cup
Dried pulses (large)	175 g	1 cup
Grains & small pulses	200 g	1 cup

LENGTH

In the UK, we generally use centimetres (cm) to measure short lengths. If you prefer to use inches (in), use the chart below to make the conversion.

1 cm	½ inch
2.5 cm	1 inch
3 cm	1¼ inches
5 cm	2 inches
8 cm	3¼ inches
10 cm	4 inches
20 cm	8 inches
25 cm	10 inches

Index

Acknowledgements

I owe a huge thank you to my little family – you've made me the cook I am today, forever creating recipes and finding inventive ways to get you to finish your meals! So, children, when you're older and have moved out, don't ask me how to make your favourite dishes, they're all in here!

To all my Instagram friends, thank you for always giving my recipes so much love and asking how I make them, they're all in this book – I promise! It was you who convinced me that there was an appetite for a cookbook and gave me the confidence to write it!

A big thank you to my brilliant publishing team for all their hard work on the book. Amanda Harris, my literary agent at YMU, Sam Jackson, who commissioned me at Penguin Random House and Dan Hurst, who project and copy edited the book.

Thank you also to the creative team, who made everything look so beautiful. To Nikki Ellis, thank you for the lovely design. To the photographers: Yuki Sugiura, thank you for the beautiful pictures of the food; and Karis Kennedy, thank you for the gorgeous portraits. To Benjamina Ebuehi and Sonali Shah, who made the food look so beautiful, a big thank you to you both. Finally, to Maurice Flynn for styling my hair so wonderfully, Fran Abrahamovitch for the beautiful make up, and Kelly Hidge for dressing me in such gorgeous clothes. Thank you all.